An Unlikely Nur

The story of a nurse and midv

Anne Reavill

It is well over thirty five years since I last worked as a nurse and midwife, and it is only recently that I have begun to really think about it all again. This has largely been following being a patient myself in hospital and seeing just how much everything has changed since then. As I started to write the memories kept flooding back, many so vivid that they could have been yesterday. Everything I have written is true as far as I remember, although all names have been changed, as have the timing and place of certain incidents. Most patients are an amalgamation of several I have cared for, and similarly most of the nurses and midwives are not based on any one individual, but are a mixture typical of several that I have known.

Contents

I.

The beginning—why 1

'Please Nurse, can I have a bedpan?'

Was she talking to me? I looked ä
was no one else near, just a couple of n
the ward. I hesitated for a moment, v
fetch one of them. But I knew what to dc

'Yes, of course,' I replied.

I collected a metal bedpan from the
slightly by rinsing it through with warn
ward I drew the curtains around her. Sl
quite easily to sit up on the pan in bed w
the curtains. After a minute 'I'm ready N
pan and returned it to the sluice before ç
wash her hands. At this point I wasn't
knew that sometimes output needed to
recorded, so I went to find the Staff Nur
me that it could be discarded, so the par
bedpan washer and flushed, then taken ol
its place in the rack.

I was nearing the end of my preliminary
nine week course run at the appre
Preliminary Training School, or PTS as it w
a short distance from the hospital. During
weeks of training we all, that is me and the
had to spend a couple of mornings on a wä
experience in giving bed baths to real patien
the dummy we had in our classroom. We
and my fellow student, Nancy, and I had jus
task and were clearing up when this patient
with her request. With me in my brand new
she would have no way of knowing just how

was. W
happen
    'I h
myself
Nancy
    Thi
visit th
guinea
who h
tractic
to hav
above
or to
difficu
and t
espec
the sh
    O
that s
we n
such
appe
patie
and
strip
just
nake
rare
quic
wor

all
har
was

7

hen I rejoined my colleague she asked me what had
ed.

ad to give her a bedpan,' I stated, rather proud of
at having completed the task on my own initiative.
looked duly impressed.

s was only our second time on the ward. On our first
e previous week we had bathed two patients. Our first
 pig was Mrs Jordan, a sixty something year old lady
ad fallen and fractured her hip. Her leg was held in
n to help reposition the bone fragments correctly prior
ing it pinned in a day or so. She had a pulley attached
 to help her raise herself when needed, to sit up more
ull herself up the bed, but even so movement was both
lt and painful for her. We were all too aware of this
errified of causing her pain, which made us hesitant,
ially when it came to washing her back and changing
eet.

r next patient, Mrs Tippett, was a bit more mobile in
he was able to sit herself out in a chair afterwards while
ade her bed. She had a colostomy. I had never seen
 a thing before and tried not to show my feelings at its
arance. We had, of course, been taught to respect a
nt's modesty as much as possible, but she had been in
ut of hospital for some time and become quite used to
ping off in front of staff. She most probably didn't know
ow new we were to the job, but I had never seen anyone
d before, apart from my own family, and then only very
y. It was something I was going to have to get used to
kly. Perhaps it was just as well I was starting on a
en's ward.

n the way back to the PTS the others had been full of it
nd seemed to have enjoyed every moment. They could
lly wait for next time. I wasn't so sure. Of course I said it
 great, but it had really been quite a shock. How on earth

would I be able to cope with some of the things I would be sure to see, much worse than just a colostomy? Perhaps nursing was not going to be for me after all.

I was dreading our next visit to the ward the following week. Once again we had to bed bath two patients. The first was Mrs Jordan once again. By now her hip had been pinned and she could move better, even get out of bed, which made us more confident. Mrs Tippet had gone home so our second patient was someone different and we completed our task in good time. It was just after this that I was asked for the bedpan. This time on our journey back I felt quite different. I had begun to feel like a real nurse and had actually enjoyed myself—even giving the bedpan, the first of who knows how many thousands I would be giving to patients over the next three years.

Why had I decided to take up nursing? You might expect the answer to this question to be the standard 'I want to help people' and to some extent I suppose this was true. I certainly wanted to do something both interesting and worthwhile, but until recently I had never for a moment given it any consideration. At school anyone who said they wanted to be a nurse was considered by many of us to be a real goody- goody. When I left school aged just 15 the only thing I was certain about was that I did not want to train as a secretary, which was what many girls did then. Not knowing what else I wanted to do, I had rather drifted into Art College, since art was one thing I had always been good at. It was while I was there that two of my friends took holiday jobs over the summer as Nursing Auxiliaries (now known as Healthcare Assistants). They had both really enjoyed themselves and, hearing them talking about some of their experiences, it all sounded fascinating, if rather scary.

Perhaps, I thought, there was rather more in it than I had previously realised.

'Would you like to go on to train,' I asked one of them.

'Oh no,' she said. 'You earn a pittance when you train. At least you get a bit more as an auxiliary.'

'But once you're qualified you'd be better off.'

'I don't think I'd cope. The training is really hard.'

As I had left school early I didn't have any O levels, apart from art which I took when I first started at the college. O levels were then the equivalent of GCSE grade 3 or above. Because of this I assumed I wasn't qualified to train as a nurse anyway. But I had to do something and where we lived in the country there was little work available for young people other than in the few local shops or pubs, and certainly no opportunities for training for a career. So I went to the nearest Labour Exchange, now known as a Job Centre. The woman I spoke to turned out to be very helpful and one of the suggestions she made was nursing. She said I was the right age and the local hospitals were looking for suitable candidates. She went on to explain that to enter nurse training the minimum qualification was officially three subjects at O levels, although there were attempts to increase this to five. However you could be accepted if you passed an entrance test.

That was how I came to pluck up enough courage to apply and was subsequently invited for an interview. My parents accompanied me and Matron, a woman of quiet authority, interviewed me on my own, then my parents and then us all together. I still wasn't altogether sure about training. After all it took three years and I didn't really expect I would last that long, plus I would earn more as an auxiliary. I actually said this to Matron, but she just shook her head and said 'You should train' and that was that! She went on to say a bit more about the course and how by the end I would become a sensible and responsible Staff Nurse. I had never thought of myself as sensible and had never had any real responsibility in my life, so I could not imagine this at all.

Next I was introduced to one of the Sister Tutors, who took me to the classroom to sit the entrance test, which consisted of questions on simple maths and English and didn't seem at all difficult. Then it was to the sewing room to be measured up for uniform in the hope that it would be needed. And that was it. A few days later I had a letter saying that I had passed the entrance test and had been accepted to start in January with the next intake of new students.

January 1963. That winter was one of the worst on record; certainly the worst I have known, either before or since. For the previous month we had been snowed up at home where I lived on the border of Dartmoor with my parents and younger sister. The snow was at least two feet deep—more where it had drifted—and after a while it had frozen hard, so hard that you could walk on top, although every so often it would give way and you would sink to above your knees.

The day I was due to start my nurse training was the first day we were able to escape, and my parents took me by car to Torquay, some 30 miles away. The roads were passable by now, but very icy, so we had chains put on the car wheels to prevent slipping. As we neared the town the roads gradually cleared so that we clanked along on the now unnecessary chains. We were in good time, which was just as well because there was a list of items that I still needed to buy before starting, not having been able to get to a town to shop. The list included a plain navy cardigan, a nurse's watch with a second hand, a bath towel, safety pins, white hair grips and some sensible plain black lace up shoes. Unfortunately I was suffering from extremely painful chilblains on my heels and toes as a result of the cold. We had no central heating at home, (virtually nobody did in those days) so my hands and feet were almost constantly cold. I'd been living in soft slippers most of the time, so these new shoes were not exactly comfortable.

On arrival at the PTS, a large and impressive Georgian house, we were greeted by Sister White, one of the two Sister Tutors who ran the preliminary course. She was a quietly spoken, grey haired woman dressed in her navy uniform with a frilly nurse's hat. She showed us all up to what was to be my room for the next nine weeks. It was a good sized single room and also beautifully warm, since the whole building was centrally heated. Quite a luxury! My chilblains were to disappear within a couple of days and I have never had one since.

Here I was left to say my farewells to my family. Waving them off I began to feel pangs of homesickness. I unpacked my few belongings and had a peak at the contents of a large flat box lying on the bed. It contained my uniform, a couple of plain grey dresses, white aprons and caps. Next to it was a navy blue cape with scarlet lining and ties, which l tried on and admired myself in the mirror. I was just wondering what to do next when Sister White knocked on my door to suggest that I came downstairs to meet the others before supper, which would be ready soon. I followed her down to the sitting room where I joined three other girls waiting there. One of the girls, tall with dark hair and a lovely smile, spoke.

'Hello, I'm Pat,' she said, 'and this Nancy, and Diane.'

The other two murmured their hellos and I introduced myself. Nancy was shorter than Pat with mousy hair and glasses making her rather serious looking, although, as I was to discover, she had a subtle sense of humour. Diane was a pretty blond who I thought looked rather bored, but perhaps that was just because she was nervous.

'Have you had to come far?' Pat asked.

I told them about my journey. 'How about you? Has the snow been bad where you live?'

'Oh, we've only come down from the Nurses Home, although none of us live very far away. We've all been working in the hospital as cadets for the last year.'

'A cadet—what's that?' I had never heard of this. It turned out that you could work in the hospital as a nursing cadet to fill in the time until you were eighteen and able to start training.

'We weren't allowed to do anything with the patients though,' Pat went on. We just worked in various departments, like Path Lab and X-ray, generally fetching and carrying. Plus we had a day release to go to the Tech, mainly studying anatomy and physiology. What have you been doing?'

I had spent two years at Art College, I told them, two years that I'd really enjoyed. Much of the previous summer had seen me with my sketch book wandering around Exeter in a long jumper and jeans plus bare feet, which for some reason had been the thing then. But I had come to realise that I would prefer to keep art as a hobby rather that make it my career.

'And since then, for the last few months, I've been working near home helping to look after horses at a pony stud.' I had enjoyed this too, but it certainly wasn't something that I wanted to do for very long. It had been hard work, but I got quite a few opportunities to ride, exercising the horses, which I loved.

There was a slight pause as they thought about this.

'Well,' said Nancy, 'if you can muck out stables you should be able to cope with nursing.'

Sister White appeared at that point. 'Supper is ready for you now if you would all like to come to the dining room,' she said. 'There's only one more of you and she has just arrived.

She'll be down in a minute. You're a very small set this time; just five of you.'

Just five of us! I could hardly believe it. The others were a bit surprised as well. An intake could be up to as many as for fourteen students, Pat told me later, although the usual number was nearer eight or nine. The hospital itself was quite small for a training school, just two hundred and something beds, but this being a holiday area, with all the extra patients this provided, it was considered that students got a wide enough experience. Also, as I had been told at my interview, a new hospital was about to be built and expected to be completed within the next five years—not soon enough for any of us to benefit from though.

We all went through and sat down to a meal of cold meat and salad that was awaiting us, not that I was at all hungry. A minute or two later the final member of our set arrived looking rather breathless.

Hello,' she said. 'I'm Hilary. I hope I haven't held you up. I thought I would never get here. My car wouldn't start and I had to get someone from the garage.'

'You've got a car,' I was impressed.

'Yes. Well I need it where I live to get to work.'

'What've you been doing?' Pat asked.

'Secretarial work. I did a secretarial course and have worked for about three years, but it was so boring and I really wanted to do something a bit more worthwhile. I've thought about nursing for ages and finally plucked up courage to do it.'

'How old are you?' Pat was always direct with her questions.

'Twenty one.' That seemed so mature to us eighteen year olds.

'I've seen you before,' said Nancy. 'Haven't you been working at the hospital?'

'Yes, I was too late applying to get into the last set, so I've been on Women's Surgical for the last couple of months, working as an auxiliary.'

'With Sister Lamb! How did you get on with her?'

Hilary laughed. 'Not too badly. I've survived anyway.'

This was the first I had heard of Sister Lamb, who sounded ominous. I now realised that I was the only one completely new to the hospital and I listened attentively to their conversation as they mentioned various goings on and people there.

That first night I lay awake for a while wondering what on earth I had let myself in for and whether I was doing the right thing. Three years seemed an interminably long period of time and I didn't really believe I would last that long. However it would be good experience and perhaps after a year or so I would think of something else I would prefer to do. In the meantime would I be able to keep up with all the studying? As for working on the wards and dealing with seriously ill patients, to say nothing of the terrifying ward sisters, how would I ever be able to cope with that?

2.

Preliminaries

The following morning we were awakened by Sister White knocking on our bedroom doors. After breakfast we were all expected to be in the classroom dressed in our uniforms. It felt strange putting on the grey serge dress and starched apron that had been provided. This was where the safety pins that had been on our list came in. They were used to hold up the apron bib. Along with this we had to wear black seamed stockings and the plain laced shoes. The white hair grips were for holding on our caps. The cap posed some problems. It was much too large when I folded it into shape, that is much too tall and not at all like the ones that I had seen nurses wearing before. Hilary helped me out here.

'You have to fold a bit of it under,' she said, giving me a demonstration and refolding the cap I had previously attempted. This looked much better and I took it from her thankfully. 'It could also do with a bit more starch,' she added. 'Most of us re-starch them when they come back from the laundry. They stay in shape much better then.'

Soon we were all sitting rather self consciously in the classroom. We now all had to address each other as 'Nurse so-and-so' and had been given name badges to pin on our dresses just above the apron. No Christian names were allowed when on duty, and that included the classroom. Most of our lectures were given by another Sister Tutor, Sister James, who ran the PTS course. She was rather severe looking with short dark hair and a round face accentuated by round rimmed glasses to match. She rarely smiled but was a good teacher, though I later wondered if she was becoming bored with teaching the same basic material every three months. Now she looked us over carefully and seemed reasonably satisfied with our appearance. At least she made no comment. They were very strict about our appearance then. Hair had to be off the collar and the length of dresses should reach to thirteen inches from the ground, regardless of how tall you were. Makeup wasn't exactly banned, but should not be too obvious. Later I quite often wore a bit of eye shadow, but kept it to a minimum and no one ever said anything. However we were told to avoid perfumes, which surprised me at first, but I learnt that the smell could be nauseating to someone feeling unwell.

Our first lecture I remember well. It was on 'cells and tissues', starting with the very basics of the anatomy and physiology we would be studying over our first year. We had lectures on the subject every morning after that. Sitting in the classroom my gaze would often wander to the skeleton hanging in the corner and to the large posters that adorned the walls depicting such things as the positions of all the muscles in the body, both male and female reproductive systems and some of the other organs. There seemed so much to learn, but I found the subject fascinating. Other lectures included nutrition and principles of nursing.

Pat, or should I say Nurse Price, was always ready with questions at lectures and, unlike me, never afraid of saying the wrong thing, which certainly enlivened things a bit. Hilary, or Nurse Steele, also spoke up from time to time, but the rest of us tended to maintain our silence unless asked anything directly. Most of our evenings were taken up with studying and preparing essays, and every couple of weeks or so we had short tests on what we had covered so far. Nancy (Nurse Hart) turned out to be the star here, almost unfailingly with the highest marks, but the rest of us seemed to be doing alright. I was just glad I was keeping up.

Much of the day was taken up with learning practical skills. There was a room set up with a hospital bed and dummy, plus basic nursing equipment. There was bed making, starting with learning how to strip the bed by folding the sheets and blankets in three and placing them over two chairs placed back to back at the foot of the bed. We then remade it, practising how to tuck in sheets and blankets using 'hospital corners'. Across the middle of the bed over the bottom sheet we placed first a rubber sheet and over this the draw sheet. This sheet was much wider than the bed and most of it was tucked in one side. The idea was that it could then be drawn through so that the patient had a clean and fresh bit to lie on, which was much easier than changing the bottom sheet and supposedly saved on laundry. When a bed was empty we were told not to tuck in the top bedclothes at the bottom, but to fold them back at the foot of the bed. Once the bed was occupied, here by the dummy, they were tucked in and we had to fold a pleat in at the bottom before tucking them in so as to allow movement and avoid pressure on the toes. Is this ever done anywhere nowadays?

Then there was the bed bath. The dummy must have been absolutely spotless, repeatedly washed by pairs of us in turn. Almost every day for the first few weeks a different pair of us carried out this procedure. One of the main problems is to prevent the patient getting cold, something not always achieved, as I know now only too well from my own more recent experiences on the receiving end as a hospital patient. We used special 'bath blankets', which were flannelette sheets, in which we wrapped patients. As well as being warm they were also slightly absorbent, so helped in drying off when we weren't as efficient as we should have been. We also learnt how to wash a patient's hair in bed, a complicated procedure which involved moving the whole mattress plus patient down over the bottom of the bed by a couple of feet, and then putting the wash bowl above them on the bed springs.

I was relieved to find that we only used the dummy to practice on. I had heard rumours of student nurses having to practice procedures on each other. Thankfully this wasn't so here. The only procedures we practised on each other were taking temperatures, pulses and respiration rates, (known as TPRs) and blood pressures. Temperatures were quite straight forward. We used glass mercury thermometers, and were warned of the dangers of them breaking in the mouth. Children and anyone who might be a bit confused should have temperatures taken under their arm, or rectally for babies. The worry seemed to be mainly focused on the dangers of glass rather than swallowing mercury, which is now known to be potentially extremely toxic, but that didn't seem to be fully appreciated then.

Taking pulses required a bit of practice, but wasn't too difficult and we could practice on ourselves at almost any time. Respiration rates were also straightforward, although were best recorded without the patient being aware. It is quite difficult to breathe naturally if you start thinking about what you are doing. Blood pressure was rather more tricky. After pumping up the blood pressure cuff you listen with a stethoscope to the artery in the crook of the elbow. You then slowly release the pressure and note the pressure at which the pulse is first heard. This is the systolic pressure and is the pressure in the artery as the heart contracts. As the pressure is reduced further the sound changes from a hard to a much softer one before fading away. This point is the background pressure in the artery between heart beats. Contrast this with today, where blood pressure is recorded automatically along with the pulse rate. Blood oxygen saturation is also usually recorded at the same time via a device attached to a finger.

Temperatures are generally recorded within seconds with an automatic probe inserted in the ear!

Then there were the fluid balance charts. For some patients it is important to record accurately both their fluid intake and output so that you can make certain they are receiving enough fluid and check their kidney function. This sounds quite straightforward, but we discovered that the hospital had just gone metric. This was in 1963, over fifty years ago, and it never ceases to amaze me that in this country we have still not completely converted to the metric system. At the time it was completely new to all of us, as at school we had only been taught the imperial system. Now we had to learn how to convert everything from pints to litres and millilitres (ml). A cup of tea would be 180ml and a pint of blood 560ml.

Other procedures we learnt included how to prepare someone for an operation and post operative care, giving injections, testing urine, simple first aid and how to give mouth to mouth resuscitation, practiced on a dummy. Injections were what worried me the most. I had a horror of receiving them myself and even the sight of needles made me want to cringe, so I wasn't sure how I would manage when the time came for me to actually have to give one myself to a live patient. Still, for the time being that seemed a long way ahead.

Even so our time at PTS soon drew to a close. During the final week we had an exam which it was essential to pass in order to be able to continue training, although one retake was permitted. On the final day the results were posted on the notice board; we had all passed. I was relieved to find I was keeping up well with the others as we all had good marks.

Also on the notice board were our ward placements. There would be no more studying for the next 3 months, just ward work. We would become very much an essential part of workforce, not 'supernumerary', as student nurses are today, where they work under the supervision of a mentor, who is one of the regular nursing staff on the ward in which they are placed. After about 3 months, though, we would start having one study day a week for three months and at the end of the year a couple of weeks full time study block. This was to be the pattern for each year, plus numerous exams on the way.

We crowded round trying to read the list.

'I'm on Men's Surgical.' Pat was delighted. 'I'll be next door to you Nancy. You're staying on Women's Surgical.'

And I'm going to Men's Medical,' said Hilary. 'That's good. I was looking forward to working there. Diane, you're on Women's Medical.'

'Where am I?' I asked, as I couldn't see past Pat.

'You're on Gynae,' she said.

I was no wiser. 'Where?'

'Gynae,' she said again. 'You're lucky. It's really nice and Sister Lessing is lovely.'

I was still not sure what she meant but didn't want to show my ignorance, so I went to my room to look at my nursing dictionary. This explained it. Gynae was short for gynaecology, or diseases of women. That was where I was to spend my first weeks gaining practical nursing experience.

3.

On the wards

Our new accommodation was in the Nurses Home attached to the hospital. All student nurses had to be resident for their first year of training. Our rooms here were typical of those for students at this time, small, with a bed down one side, a hand basin, small desk and wardrobe. Pat and Nancy, however, had opted to share a room as they had shared at PTS and found they got on well together. When I saw their room I thought they were really on to a good thing. It was large and positioned at the front of the building with views out across the front of the hospital and beyond. My room in contrast was at the back and looked out onto a hedge.

Our working week was 48 hours over five and a half days. There were early shifts, late shifts and split shifts, which could vary in length. An early shift lasted from 7.30am to 4.30pm and late shifts from 1 to 10pm. Split shifts had the afternoon free and finished at either 8 or 10pm, which made for a long day and wasn't good when followed by an early morning the next day. It was usual to have your half day before your day off and follow this by a late shift so that it was possible to go away for two nights if you wished. Later that year our hours were reduced and then we only had to work 5 days and had two whole days off every week, much appreciated by me as it meant slightly fewer early starts.

Getting up in the morning was not my strongest point. We were woken up at about 6.45am by Night Sister going round knocking loudly on our doors, so no need for an alarm. I still remained in bed until the last possible moment, washing and dragging on my uniform in a few minutes before rushing to breakfast. I rarely had time to eat any.

Breakfast was served for us in the hospital dining room and about 5 minutes before we were due on duty Night Sister arrived to call out the register to see if everyone was present who should be. If anyone was missing she would have to go back to the Nurses Home to see if they were alright or had just overslept.

Pat was right; Gynae was a good place to start. It was much smaller than Women's Surgical where I had been with Nancy to practice bed baths during PTS, and the pace of work rather more relaxed. The main Gynae ward had just 14 beds. Being on the top floor the sides of the ceiling sloped into the eves so that it didn't appear as high as it did in the larger wards. Between each bed there was a window with a radiator below. As well as this there was a 4 bedded side ward and one single room.

Sister Lessing greeted me as I arrived at 7.30am sharp to work an early shift. She was quite young compared to the sisters I had met so far, dark haired and attractive. All the staff were gathered in the office, where the nurse who had been on the previous night gave us the report and handed over for the day. She went through each patient in turn, saying what they were in for and reported what sort of night they had had and any treatment or drugs given. Most of this meant nothing to me. When this was finished Sister handed me over to Staff Nurse George to show me around and what to do.

Before starting in the ward Staff Nurse showed me a bit about how things were organized in the office. First there was the Kardex, which was a sort of flip up file. Each section held a card with patient's details summarised and it was where we recorded all nursing care and treatment. Then there was the off duty rota; very important. The rota for each week was put up about the middle of the week before. Staff Nurse also showed me the book where we could request any days off we particularly needed, such as for a dental appointment. Unless there was a really valid reason there was no guarantee your request would be granted. After that we went into the ward to begin work. The rest of the day was a whirl of bed making and baths, taking TPRs and serving drinks and meals. The time flew. By 4.30 I was exhausted and all too glad to get off duty.

It all seemed very confusing and I wondered if I would ever get the hang of it all and know what I was doing. There was always so much to remember. We always took careful notes during the report when we came on duty, writing on scraps of paper that we kept with us to refer to during the day. Most of the morning was taken up with making beds and giving bed baths. After their wash some patients might be sat out of bed and made comfortable in a chair. If it was the first day after their operation they could be very sore and need quite a bit of help and encouragement. I would run baths for those who were able to have one, and afterwards it was my job to clean the bathtub thoroughly ready for the next patient.

Meals were served from a large heated trolley that was brought up to the ward bringing breakfast, lunch and supper. In the top there were half a dozen large containers, one each for potatoes, vegetables and perhaps a meat stew for example at lunch time. In the bottom section there might be a jam sponge for pudding, with custard in one of the top containers. There was no choice of menu and no individual meals, but I don't remember anyone complaining. It was extremely rare for a patient to request a special diet, only very occasionally a vegetarian. Meals were usually served by the senior nurse on duty. I had to make sure all patients were sitting up ready with their bed table clear or sat at the table set in the centre of the ward. I then helped to hand out their meals.

Hot drinks were served at mid-morning, tea time and in the evening. The ward domestic helped to prepare the trolley that we took round and she washed up afterwards. The ward domestics were very much part of the ward team and often ruled over the kitchen with iron fisted authority. Woe betides anyone leaving it untidy or with unwashed crockery for her to find when she came on duty. We junior nurses often went in as much trepidation of them as we did the ward sisters.

The afternoons and evenings were less busy. After lunch there was an hour's quiet period before visiting from 2−4pm. Visitors often brought in flowers and I would spend much of this time hunting for vases to arrange them in, then finding spaces to put them on bedside lockers or window sills. In the evenings there were suppers to serve, followed by more visiting, then evening drinks and making sure everything was up to date before the night staff came on duty.

The sickest patient on the ward when I started was Mrs Endicott, a woman in her mid fifties. She had been admitted for a hysterectomy for cancer of the uterus (womb), but when she was opened up the cancer had spread too far and was inoperable. There were no such things as sophisticated scans available then that could be used to detect this beforehand and ordinary X-rays were not sensitive enough, so the only way to find out the severity of the cancer was to open up the abdomen and look. Now she was very frail, just skin and bone. We had to change her position regularly to prevent her from developing pressure sores, a particular danger with someone so frail. These can develop when the circulation to an area is cut off by lying in one position for too long. They are considered to be the result of bad nursing care, but can be very difficult to prevent in some cases. Every week a form had to be filled in for every ward listing anyone who had developed a sore. This went to matron's office. She would then want to know why it had happened and what was being done about it.

Mrs Endicott also had to have a catheter to drain her urine as she was unable to go to the toilet herself and I learnt how to empty the bag, measure the output and record this on her fluid balance chart. She was too weak to get out of bed and I helped wash her and change her bed, rolling her onto her side to change the sheets. I was also able to watch Staff Nurse do her dressing; not very pleasant but good experience. A few days after I started there it was apparent that her wound wasn't healing well and she was moved to a different ward where she was able to be nursed in a single room. A couple of weeks later we heard that she had died. It was sad, but in many ways I felt relieved for her. She must have suffered so much, although of course she had been given plenty of painkillers. I wasn't sure how I was ever going to get used to that sort of thing, or if I ever would.

There were usually three or four of us on duty in the mornings, but in the afternoons and evenings there were often just two. Staff Nurse George was the only fully qualified nurse apart from Sister. The most senior student was Nurse Mulligan, who was in her third year and due to take her final exams at the end of the summer. She often had to take charge of the ward for afternoons or evenings when either the Sister or Staff Nurse had their days off, which seemed to me to be a big responsibility. She had just got engaged and was very proud of her ring, which she showed to me. We weren't allowed to wear jewellery of any kind, so she wore it on a chain around her neck and tucked in to her dress.

'When are you getting married?' I asked her one evening when we were on together.

'In September,' she said, 'as soon as I have taken my finals.'

'Will you be staying on here?'

'No, my boyfriend has just started a new job near Bristol, so I will probably look for something there once we are settled. But of course we may just start a family. Who knows?'

It is hard to believe now, but many women chose not to work outside the home once they were married. They expected to be supported by their husband. It seemed a shame that after undergoing three years training someone wouldn't want to make use of it, although of course most of our nurse training was based on experienced gained while actually working on the wards. The running of the hospital was totally dependent on us students to maintain staffing levels.

During quiet spells, such as during visiting, I was sometimes able to study the patient's notes. The notes were filed in slots in a special trolley and each slot had the patient's name and their consultant written by it. It was good to sit down for a bit, so I took these opportunities to learn more about the patients eagerly. Some had had hysterectomies carried out for any of a number of reasons such as cancer or fibroids. Others had repairs of prolapses, where the uterus drops down and in severe cases can even protrude from the vagina. This occurs as a result of childbirth, especially if delivery is prolonged.

Several women came in to be sterilized after completing their families, but one of them, a Mrs Williams, had been sterilized at the young age of just 22 years. To do this the fallopian tubes, which lead from the ovaries to the uterus, are cut so as to prevent eggs travelling down them to where they could become fertilized. This was an abdominal operation; no keyhole surgery then. Mrs Williams was only recently married, but had a congenital heart defect and it wasn't considered safe for her to have children. I wondered if she and her new husband had really wanted a family, but never felt I could ask her that. It must have been a difficult decision.

As well as routine operations there were occasional emergency admissions. These were often women in early pregnancy who were bleeding and threatening to miscarry, known as threatened abortions. One day I took a bedpan from one of these patients and when I looked in it I found a small and perfectly formed foetus. In those days no actual abortions were carried out as it was still illegal.

Another day we had an emergency admission of a young woman who had developed severe abdominal pain. She was known to be a few weeks pregnant and it was suspected that she had an ectopic pregnancy. This is where the fertilized egg fails to travel all the way through the fallopian tubes to the uterus. It becomes lodged within the tube where foetus starts to develop, but unfortunately there is no room for it to grow much and the pressure causes increasingly severe pain. This is an emergency from which a patient may die if it is not recognised and treated quickly because the tube will eventually burst, causing severe internal bleeding. This patient was taken quickly to theatre where the affected tube, which was on the verge of rupturing, was removed. It was her first pregnancy and she had been so looking forward to having her baby. Luckily women have two fallopian tubes, one from each ovary, so she would still be fertile. I had never realised so much could go wrong with the process of reproduction and was amazed at just how much some women had to go through.

4.

Operating day

The weekly routine revolved around 'operating day'. Patients would be admitted the afternoon before the operation. This was partly, I was told, to give them time to get used to the ward, but also for them to be checked by a doctor. They would need to have various blood tests and blood cross matched ready in case it was needed.

On operating day there was a very different atmosphere in the ward. Everyone was quieter than usual as patients were prepared for their surgery. They were told to have a bath, and then donned theatre gowns and a cloth cap to cover their hair. We had to check that they were not wearing any makeup or jewellery. If they wanted to keep on their wedding rings we covered them with tape. Any valuables were put in a locked cupboard in the office. About half an hour to an hour before they were due to go down to theatre they were given a premed, which would usually be omnopon, an opiate, to make them relaxed and drowsy, sometimes together with scopolamine, which reduces secretions, making the mouth dry but reducing the chance of vomiting. Then they were left with their curtains drawn until the theatre porter came with a trolley to collect them. One of us always accompanied them and stayed in the anaesthetic room until they were asleep under anaesthetic.

Once their operation was over and they were ready to return to the ward, someone from theatre would call us and one of us would go down to collect the patient. On return to the ward they would still not be round from their anaesthetic and would have an airway in place. There were no such things as recovery wards then, where nowadays patients stay after surgery until fully conscious and stable. My job would be to stay in the ward with patients until they were round, the first signs of which were gagging on the airway and trying to spit it out. Even after this someone had to remain in the ward at all times, and that usually meant me. There was still a lot to do. There were recordings, such a pulse and blood pressure, which might need taking at least every 15 minutes at first until we were sure the patient's condition was stable. Understandably I was nervous to begin with, but Staff Nurse George showed me exactly what to do. If I was worried about anything someone more experienced was always near at hand and I soon took it all in my stride.

When they first came round from their anaesthetics patients who had undergone an abdominal operation often seemed to be in a good deal of pain, which always worried me. They were very quickly given an injection of a strong painkiller, usually pethidine. Two people always had to check these sorts of drugs, known as DDAs which stands for Dangerous Drugs Act, the act which controls how they are administered, stored and recorded. One of the two of you had to be a registered nurse or doctor, but I was often the second person checking the prescription with them and signing the record book. It was then also my responsibility to check that it was given to the correct patient and witness its administration.

Then there were the intravenous infusions, or drips as they are known. We had to work out how many drops per minute they needed to run and set them at this rate. Control was by a clamp attached to the tubing, and was a lot more difficult to achieve than it sounds. You could get it running just right, but while you were doing something else the patient would move their arm so that when you next checked it was either going too fast or too slow and need readjusting. Worse still they sometimes were found to have stopped completely with the result that the cannula (the needle through which the fluid was running) had become blocked. Much time was then spent milking the tube to push fluid through and get it going again.

Sometimes patients would need oxygen for a while. Oxygen cylinders were kept at the end of the ward and could be wheeled to the bedside. I was a bit nervous of handling them knowing they contained gas at such high pressure. To turn them on first there was a main valve that hissed loudly when opened. Then there was another valve which acted to regulate the flow. When in use we had to check their gauge regularly and call the porters to bring up new cylinders to replace them when they were getting low. As well as this there was the suction apparatus which needed to be kept nearby. This could be vital for clearing the airways of an unconscious patient should they become blocked. The area around a bed could become quite cluttered. Nowadays all beds would have both piped oxygen and suction making things much easier.

Another thing I found was that patients often felt very cold after their return to the ward. The operating theatres always seemed warm to people working there, but they wore gowns and masks over their clothes. Patients would only be covered with sterile cotton towels, just exposing the area to be operated on, so it wasn't surprising that they felt so cold afterwards. I would then get them a hot water bottle. These had to be prepared very carefully according to a set procedure that we had learnt at PTS. The water had be a certain temperature, not too hot, and this was prepared in a jug. To fill the bottle we first had to expel the air, and then fill it using a funnel and pouring in the water from the jug. Finally we put a cover over the bottle. We were constantly warned of the dangers of a patient getting burnt. Some patients might be too weak to move much or drowsy due to the drugs they had been given, also making them less aware of pain. I remember one instance later in my training when a patient did get a small burn from a hot water bottle leading to blistering on the skin. The nurse who had given her the bottle was hauled up in front of Matron. Nowadays no hot water bottles are allowed in hospital at all, which in many ways is a shame as they can be so comforting, but I suppose the risk of being sued if anyone got burnt is so great that they just can't take the risk. The compensation culture has a lot to answer for.

One operating day when I had been there about a month we had a shorter than usual list. I was preparing to take a patient down to theatre, doing the various checks necessary, when Sister took me to one side.

'Would you like to stay down in theatre with her and watch the operation?' she asked. 'We aren't too busy here today, so we can spare you.'

'Oh, yes please,' I said, jumping at the opportunity, at the same time feeling nervous at the prospect. I didn't want to make a fool of myself there by fainting or anything.

Down in theatre the patient was soon anaesthetized and wheeled into theatre. Theatre Sister showed me where to get a gown and mask to wear before going in myself. I stood well back, afraid of getting in the way. Everyone seemed very busy at first getting things organized, but then suddenly they were ready to start. As the surgeon made the first incision I tried not to look too closely, but as he went on I forced myself to watch and soon became fascinated by it all.

After going through the skin there was a thick layer of fat before entering the abdominal cavity itself. She was suffering from fibroids, which are large muscular growths that develop in the wall of the uterus, and I was amazed at their size. The poor woman must have felt as though she was heavily pregnant all the time. Afterwards I went back to the ward with her and stayed with her during her initial recovery. It was a great experience for me and I felt it gave me a better understanding of what the patients were going through.

Another patient I remember well was Mrs Lawson. She came in for a very big operation, a pelvic exenteration. This I learnt was the removal of all organs from within the pelvis; that is uterus, much of the colon and bladder, which would leave her with a double colostomy. This type of operation wasn't often done, but she had cervical cancer that had already spread to the adjacent organs and it was her only hope of survival. Due to the seriousness of her operation the single side ward was prepared for her.

She came in with her family, her husband and daughter. She was a lovely woman, only in her late forties, and seemed resigned to what was to come. Her daughter turned out to be a student nurse at another hospital and she was understandably upset and worried about her mother. Apparently she later told Nurse Mulligan that if anything happened to her mother she would give up nursing.

I had relatively little to do with Mrs Lawson's care, as this was carried out by the more experienced staff. They were all subdued as they discussed her progress following her operation.

'After she came round the first thing she said was 'It's all over'' Staff Nurse told us. 'But it's really just beginning.'

This was, I discovered, very true. She did not make good progress. I helped Staff Nurse get her out of bed a few days after the operation, and was shocked to find how weak she was still. She could barely stand her own weight for even a few seconds as we got her out of bed to her in a chair. Over the next few days her condition continued to deteriorate and her family were allowed extra time to visit. After I came back from my days off I found out she had died.

I suppose the operation had been her only hope, but the surgery had clearly been too much for her body to cope with. The survival rate for this type of operation was low, which was one reason why it was rarely carried out. Perhaps it is better today with improved after care and treatment. There is also now a much wider range of treatments available to combat cancer, such as chemotherapy, which might have at least extended her life.

At the beginning of every week a notice was put up on the board in the Nurses Home listing students who were to move to a different ward the following week. This was known as the 'Change List'. As soon as it was posted a small crowd would gather round, everyone examining it anxiously to see if their name was there and, if so, find out where they were going to be working next. The usual length of time spent on the larger wards, such as the main medical and surgical wards, was twelve weeks, but for smaller wards and specialities like the eye ward, ear, nose and throat (ENT) and Gynae it was normally just six so that as many specialities as possible were able to be fitted into the three years training. Therefore when I started my sixth week on Gynae I knew I was due for a move.

Pat, Nancy and Hilary all seemed to be getting on well and enjoying their wards, but not so Diane. She became even quieter than usual and went back to her home whenever she could for her time off, so I rarely saw her. It was Hilary who told me how unhappy she was. On her very first day on Women's Medical someone had died and, with so many seriously ill patients, she found much of the work too upsetting. Then a few days later I met Hilary again at coffee time and she told me Diane was leaving.

'Some people just can't cope with the sort of things we have to deal with,' Hilary said. 'It often isn't easy,'

That was very true. It was something that worried me. I had had a relatively gentle introduction so far on Gynae. Although two patients had died while I was there I hadn't been directly involved with either of them at the time. But this sort of thing was not generally discussed then. I don't think any of us had heard of counselling, which we hear so much of today, although I am sure the Sister Tutors would have given us a sympathetic ear if we had turned to them. I was sorry Diane was going, but I hadn't really got to know her as well as the others. But because of her departure it was of no surprise to me when I read on the change list that I was going to Women's Medical next.

During my final week on Gynae I had to make sure my Record Book was up to date. This book, which had been given to us when we finished PTS, listed every procedure we might be expected to undertake as a nurse. It was up to us to see that everything we had done was ticked and then signed off by a Sister or Staff Nurse when they considered us proficient. Completion of this book was a requirement of the General Nursing Council (GNC) as part of our training, and it would eventually be examined by them to make certain we had received sufficient experience before becoming State Registered Nurses.

As well making sure our record book was up to date, when finishing on a ward we had the dreaded ward report. You had a meeting with the ward sister, who would discuss with you how you had got on, what you had done well and what needed improving. She wrote this up on a form for you to sign to show that you had read it and discussed it with her. The form then went to Matron as part of your record. So it was with some apprehension that I went to Sister Lessing for my first ward report. I knew I hadn't made any serious errors during my time there, but was still nervous. However I didn't need to have worried as she seemed reasonably pleased with my progress. She did say that I needed to show a bit more confidence, but that would no doubt develop with time.

5.

Life in the Nurses' Home

Our life in the Nurses' Home sounds highly restricted to anyone today, but we were also well looked after and even had some luxuries. Of course we all did sometimes want to rebel against the rules; after all we were given so much responsibility on the wards and yet off duty we felt we were being treated like children. But residence there was compulsory for our first year, after which we could move out and make our own arrangements if we wished. Most people did so sooner or later, although we could move back at any time.

The Nurses' Home was run by the Home Sister, Sister Edwards. She had an office where we were able to see her at most times during the day. There she kept the books that we had to sign if we were away for our days off or wanted a late pass. She also ran the doctor's surgery. If we wanted to see the doctor she made an appointment for us and a local GP came in most mornings. We had all had to register with him when we started our training. Sister Edwards would also dish out things like aspirin to us if we needed any for headaches or period pains. The room next to her office was kept as a Sick Bay, not just for resident staff, but also for sick non-resident students who she felt needed to be there so she could keep an eye on them.

If we had the morning or day off we put up a tab on the door of our room so that when Night Sister came round in the morning she didn't wake us up and we could sleep in. Breakfast was then served a bit later in our sitting room. We would come down for this in our dressing gowns and slippers and have a leisurely cereal, boiled eggs, toast and tea. But as well as this, once a week we were actually allowed breakfast in bed. This had to be ordered the night before. It was brought up to our rooms by one of the domestics and when finished we put the empty trays outside our doors to be collected. I would then often go back to bed until lunch, by which time I would need to get ready to go on duty if on late shift.

Other meals were all taken in the nurses' dining room in the hospital, which was set out in a series of long tables. This was for all nursing staff except the ward sisters, who had a separate, smaller dining room next door. Doctors had their own doctor's mess elsewhere in the building. All staff on duty had their meals included. The food wasn't too bad, certainly better than the school dinners I had been eating not so very long before, but never up to home standards of course. Breakfast I rarely got to in time, but between 9 and 10am there was the mid-morning break. Here every table had both a white and a brown sliced loaf, butter, a couple of different flavoured jams, lemon curd, fish paste and marmite. After a couple of hour's heavy work on the wards I was starving and tucked into all this with relish, working my way through the different fillings; not the healthiest of diets.

All this did not last. By my final year the system had changed, presumably for economic reasons, and we all had to buy meal tokens for lunch and supper. Mid-morning and afternoon breaks were reduced to tea or coffee and a few biscuits. The result was that many nurses skipped meals to save money—not ideal given the work we did.

For our uniforms we had large grey laundry boxes issued. These were collected once a week and returned clean a few days later. For our own laundry there was a room with a large sink—no washing machines then—plus a drying cupboard, ironing board and iron. I very rarely used any of these. The few things I washed were dried on the radiator in my room, but I'm afraid most of the rest was taken back home to my mother. Not that there was much. Most days I wore nothing but my uniform, only wearing mufti on evenings and days off. On a late shift I usually slept in late and on a split shift after a busy morning all I felt like doing was having a nap until time to go back on duty at tea time.

Gradually I got to know some of the other students from working with them on the wards, meeting them at meal breaks or in the evening in the Nurses Home, either in the common room or watching television. It seemed that the catchment area for the hospital was relatively small and most students came from the local area. In the course of my training we did have a couple from Scotland and Ireland, and one from Norway, which was quite unusual. It was only after I had been there about a year that we had the first two West Indian students. Also at about the same time we had two married students, both of whom had families and so of course were a bit older than the rest of us. They were even allowed to live out throughout their training, so things were beginning to become a bit more flexible.

These days I saw rather little of the others in my set unless we happened to be working on the same shift. Our days off only occasionally coincided, so mostly it was a matter of just bumping into them in the dining room. But some evenings we would congregate in Pat and Nancy's room drinking mugs of coffee, which we were able to make in a small kitchen where a good supply of milk was left out for us every evening. News of any interesting or unusual cases, and any deaths, were always circulated rapidly around the hospital grapevine, so there was always plenty for us to discuss, as well as comparing our experiences so far.

'I heard you had another death on your ward today.' Pat said to Hilary one evening.

'Yes. He'd been in for a couple days with a coronary and seemed to be doing alright, but had another really bad attack.'

'Was he old?' Pat asked.

'I think he was about sixty.' That seemed old to us then.

'You didn't have to lay him out did you?'

'Yes. I did it with Staff Nurse. But I had done that before when I was an auxiliary.'

We were all quiet for a moment in awe of this. The rest of us had yet to see a patient after death, let alone lay someone out. But it would be all part of our duties in the future.

'We've got a new Staff Nurse on our ward,' said Nancy, changing the subject. 'She trained at a London teaching hospital and is very grand. Everything we do she's telling us how it would have been done there.'

'My parents wanted me to go to London,' Pat looked a bit rueful. 'But I didn't do well enough in my O levels. It was entirely my own fault—I didn't do the work.'

To be able to train at a London teaching hospital you needed a minimum of 5 O levels to be accepted for training.

'At least you've gone ahead and started training,' I said. 'One of the girls at my school was like you, didn't get good enough O levels to get into a London hospital, so she just gave up the idea. She had wanted to be a nurse for as long as I could remember and just gave up.'

And yet here I was, I could have gone on to say, someone who never even considered nursing until recently and without O levels, doing nurse training.

'She can't have been that really interested then, just liked the idea,' said Pat, and I agreed.

'It's the same qualification, so I don't see that it makes any difference where you train,' said Nancy.

'The trouble with teaching hospitals is that you're competing with medical students for experience,' Hilary told

40

us. 'I know someone who went to one and she hardly ever got a chance to do things like dressings. Medical students even did most of the blood pressures.'

'That doesn't sound too bad to me. All I seem to do is blood pressures. My hand aches by the end of the day after pumping up the cuff all the time.'

'Well I'm really glad now that I didn't get in,' Pat went on. 'I would have had to live in for the entire three years. At least here it is only for the first year. I can't wait to move out.'

Personally I didn't mind living in too much. It was good not to have to travel in every day, and I usually went away for my days off.

We couldn't carry on talking for too long though. The front door to the Nurses' Home was locked by 11pm when the Night Sister did her rounds. By this time we were all supposed to be tucked up in our beds. If any room had a light showing under the door she would rap loudly until it was turned out. All this seems very restrictive, but we did need our night's sleep ready for our early start and I don't remember ever being disturbed.

If we wanted to stay out late after the Nurses' Home was locked, once a week we were allowed a late pass until midnight, and once a month we could get one until 1am. But we were not given a key. When we got back we had to go into the main hospital and get whoever was on the switchboard to bleep the Night Sister, who would have to come down to escort us to the Nurses' Home and let us in with instructions to be very quiet and not wake anyone. I often wondered how the Night Sister managed to fit all this in. As I discovered later, as well as having to do rounds of the hospital wards she also had charge of the Casualty Department.

If we wanted to go into town during the day we could get a bus from the stop at the bottom of the hospital drive. If we were lucky an ambulance would pass on its way back from

41

delivering someone to the hospital. If they saw any nurses waiting they would often stop and give us a lift sitting in the back. I'm sure they would not be allowed to do that today. We didn't have much to spend though. My first monthly pay check was just over £24, but that was after all deduction including board and lodgings, so I didn't find it too bad.

A couple of times a year we would have a party, held in a separate building behind the Nurses' Home. But no men were allowed in the Nurses' Home, ever. I remember on one occasion on the night of one of our parties the weather was atrocious, with torrential rain. Someone actually allowed some men through the Nurses' Home after they had parked their car in front, to avoid them getting too wet. Somehow the Assistant Matron found out (she was probably keeping a discrete eye on proceedings) and she was nearly apoplectic.

We were never short of men at these parties. I am not sure how most of them were invited or got to hear about it, although for some reason the doctors rarely attended. We had essentially no contact with them outside work, contrary to popular belief. I met a young policeman at one party and went out a few times afterwards. When he came to the Nurses' Home he was only allowed as far as the porch, where he would have to wait for someone to fetch me if I was not there already.

I also went out a few times with a young curate. He was the son of friends of my parents and his first job was a parish near the hospital. As he was new to the area and didn't know anyone we met up a few times. However I had no intention of settling down yet and there was no way I was going to be a vicar's wife, so this did not last long. I did manage to introduce him to a couple of other nurses though, and a few years later he married one of the staff nurses there.

We also often received invitations for other events which would be posted on the notice board. If you were interested you went to see Matron's secretary who organised it all. Quite often the local theatre would offer half a dozen tickets; perhaps if the current production wasn't selling well and they wanted to fill up a few more seats. Nancy and I took these up a couple of times when we were both off duty together. Another time Hilary and I went to a much grander do, a dinner at the Royal Naval College in Dartmouth. Hilary drove us there and we had a wonderful time. We were the only ones who took up the invitation, which surprised me.

Although this may sound as though we had a lively social life, as often as not I spent evenings off just watching television. In those days there were only two channels, BBC and ITV and where I lived at home we could only get BBC, so ITV was new to me. I was able to watch programs I had only ever heard of before, like Coronation Street, for the first time. I also remember watching the first ever broadcast of 'Top of the Pops' on BBC, which I thought was fantastic. It was the first time I had seen any of the popular groups that I knew from the radio actually on television. Of course we worked up to as late as 10pm two or three evenings a week and I usually went home for my days off, so there weren't all that many free evenings. But some of the other nurses didn't seem to go out at all. Perhaps they were just too exhausted after work. There was also always the problem of getting evenings off just when you wanted them and at the same time as your friends.

6.

All change

Women's Medical was a large traditional Nightingale style ward with rows of beds lined up along either side. It was high ceilinged with tall sash windows which, since there was no double glazing then, would have made it cold if it wasn't for the powerful radiators in front of each of them. A lot of their heat must have been wasted. The tops of these windows could be opened if the weather was warm enough and we had a long pole with a hook on the end to reach up to the catch. There was also one single room situated between this and Men's Medical next door and this could be used by either ward. In practice the room rarely seemed to be used except when a member of staff or perhaps a local doctor was admitted. It was one of the few perks of the job I suppose.

It was very much an acute medical ward. Many of the patients would today be admitted to intensive care or coronary care units, but we had none of these then, although they were just beginning to be introduced in larger hospitals. The average patient's age must have been around twice that of those in Gynae and they were admitted with a wide range of conditions including heart attacks, strokes, diseases of the blood such as leukaemia and overdoses. We didn't get any medical lectures until our second year, so it was all very confusing at first. It was with much trepidation that I started my first day's work there, unsure how I would cope with caring for such seriously ill patients. But I soon got caught up in the busy routine of work where there was little time to think of anything else.

Sister Rowland ran the ward assisted by two Staff Nurses. Staff Nurse Norland, the senior of the two, had worked there for years and seemed to take me under her wing at first, taking time to explain the patient's conditions and the care and treatment they needed. Perhaps she did this for all newcomers. There were several other students, including Kay Sergeant, a friendly girl I had already met and chatted to on occasions at meal times. She was in her second year and we soon became friends.

The routine here was to give full bed baths to patients on alternate sides of the ward each day so that they were all bathed every other day. Those who could get up were helped to the bath and those not having baths had washes, often referred to as a 'top and tail', given by the night staff.

As well as the routine bed baths and washes, on this ward we had the ritual known as the 'back round', carried out every four hours on patients who were bed bound to prevent them developing bed sores. That was most of the patients here. Pressure areas, i.e. the sacral area, elbows and heels, were massaged with either cream or powder, made clean and dry and the patient's position changed. Then there was the bedpan round. Bedpans were warmed slightly by rinsing them with warm water, then loaded onto a trolley and taken round the ward, offering one to each patient—by which time the bedpans were usually cold again. This was done at regular intervals, such as after meals and just before visiting hours.

We worked in pairs almost all the time since most of the work required two of us to move patients, lifting them up the bed or helping them into a chair when they were unsteady on their feet. It was heavy work, with none of the hoists that are used today to help us. We had been instructed in the way to lift patients at PTS and it was drummed into us regularly that we should never ever attempt to lift anyone on our own. Even so we would sometimes do such things as sitting people up on our own if there was no one else near at hand, which meant sitting them forward, pulling out the backrest and rearranging the pillows. Luckily obesity wasn't the problem that it is now, but it was still heavy work. It wasn't surprising that a lot of nurses had bad backs.

One consequence of this regular movement from patient to patient as we moved around the ward was the risk of cross infection. We were reminded regularly of the importance of hand washing between patients, especially when doing the back rounds. The problem with this was that it often meant having to walk the length of the ward to the wash basin, which was at one end near the entrance. One way around this was to carry a wash bowl for us to use on the trolley and change the water after every few patients. Even so it was not ideal. As well as that there were communal wash bowls and bedpans. The plastic wash bowls were cleaned thoroughly and bedpans put through a wash cycle in the hob designed for the purpose, but none were actually sterilized between patients. Many people criticize current standards of cleanliness in hospitals, but at least all patients have individual bowls and bedpans with disposable inserts, which must be an improvement.

Another major problem was the availability of fresh laundry. We usually had barely enough to just cover making up clean beds following a patient's discharge, let alone change sheets for anybody else. Using draw sheets meant that they could be pulled through so there was a clean patch to sit on, but often we could only change linen if it was actually soiled. We often complained to the laundry, but their excuse was that it couldn't be done any quicker and they even told us that we changed sheets too often, unnecessarily. This problem was not specific to our hospital, as I discovered later. I don't really know why there was always such a difficulty—perhaps there was just not enough linen to start with—but the practice nowadays seems to be to change sheets daily, so laundry problems must have been sorted somehow. Seeing that most patients are in bed for a large part if not all of the day, this must be important in reducing hospital acquired infections.

The pace of work here was certainly greater than I was used to, with many patients unable to do anything for themselves and thus needing total nursing care. We were on the go every minute of the day; indeed this was expected of us and even when it was a bit quieter, such as during visiting, we could never look as though we had nothing to do. There were still a lot of jobs that we were able to catch up on during these times. There was general tidying up, mainly the sluice. The draw macs, the rubber sheets that went under the draw sheets, were put into disinfectant to soak after patients were discharged and needed to be rinsed and hung over rails to dry. In the sterilization room there were drums to pack with cotton wool swabs ready to go for sterilization, which was carried out centrally in large autoclaves in a unit attached to the operating theatres. We put special tape on them that had stripes that turned dark brown when the drum reached a certain temperature to show that it had been sterilized adequately. The doctor's rubber gloves had to be washed and packed for resterilization. They had to be thoroughly dried both inside and out, and the inside powdered so that they could be put on easily. Nothing was disposable and the idea that anything could be thrown away after use seemed incredibly wasteful.

Serving meals was also a much bigger undertaking here as so many patients were on special diets. These might be diabetic, low fat, low calorie, low or high protein to name but a few. We had several patients admitted with gastric ulcers and they were given gastric diets, which were soft and low in fibre, usually something like steamed fish and mashed potato. The cause of these ulcers was then thought to be stress and too much acid in the stomach, so they were treated with bed rest and antacid medicines. It was some years later before it was discovered that gastric ulcers are often due to an infection which can be easily treated with antibiotics. For some reason special diets were served last. This always seemed illogical to me, not just because they often got cold waiting, but also because you had to remember who *not* to serve with a normal meal. There was such a fast turnover of patients there that following your days off almost half the ward could have changed, making it very difficult to remember who was supposed to have what. On more than one occasion I went to give someone their special diet only to find they had already eaten half of a normal meal. When it eventually became my job to serve meals I would give out diets first. Some patients needed feeding and this was a task I quite enjoyed, not least because it was a chance to sit down.

There were three medical consultants and each of them did a round of their patients once a week. On those days we all had to make sure the ward was tidy and their patients ready for them on time. Occasionally one of us was asked to join the round with Sister and I enjoyed doing this, finding it really interesting and learning a lot. The consultant would be accompanied by his registrar and houseman, and Sister showed him to each patient in turn, handing him the relevant notes. I helped by drawing the curtains around and back again after he had finished. Afterwards patients often would beckon to me and ask rather confidentially what was meant by something they had said and I would try to translate it into lay terms as far as I could so that they understood.

It was during my time on Women's Medical that I felt that I became confident in many basic nursing procedures. Firstly there were blood pressures. Some patients needed recordings every four hours, so there were regular blood pressure rounds to do. We had been taught that a normal blood pressure for an adult was one hundred plus their age, which meant that for an eighty year old a systolic of 180 wasn't considered all that excessive, though it is far higher than would be considered ideal today. Taking blood pressure required putting a cuff around the patients arm and pumping it up manually, which was quite hard work and my hand would ache by the time I had finished a round.

Then there was giving injections. I had given my first one while on Gynae and had been so nervous at the time, gritting my teeth as I plunged the needle in to the poor patient that had to suffer my attempt. I was still dreading just the thought of it, but this was where Sister Mortimer came in. She was a Clinical Instructor, only recently appointed, and her role complemented that of the tutors in that she worked entirely on the wards with students, moving regularly between the different wards. Being able to have individual attention like this was invaluable. She was enthusiastic about her work, having endless patience and giving encouragement when needed. Now she was on our ward for a couple of weeks and while there she decided that I was to do all injections that were due when I was on duty with her.

Since there were no disposable syringes and needles then, injections took a bit of preparation. Glass syringes and needles were kept in spirit in a shallow dish covered with a lid. When selecting a syringe shaft and plunger you had to make sure they matched up by looking at numbers with which they were all marked. If you got the wrong pairing the plunger wouldn't fit properly and might be either loose or stick. Then the needles had to be examined. After being reused a few times the point could become hooked, making them blunt and more painful when used. This was checked by wiping it down with a cotton wool swab and if it was hooked it would catch, in which case you would have to throw it away and find a new one.

With Sister Mortimer's encouragement I soon became adept at shaking down ampoules so that all the fluid was at the base and breaking them open, which meant using a small file and scratching on one side so that the top snapped off easily, then drawing up the drug and expelling any air. Injections could be either intramuscular or subcutaneous, both being a slightly different technique. Subcutaneous are, as the name implies, given just below the skin, so the skin is pinched up slightly to insert the needle. Intramuscular are given more deeply in the muscle, usually in the buttock, and here it is important to give it in the right area to avoid hitting a nerve. Mentally you have to divide the buttock into quadrants and use the upper outer area only. I was extremely nervous and slow with my first few attempts, but surprised myself by quickly mastering these techniques and soon began to feel quite confident with it all.

As a junior nurse it was inevitable that I was involved with ward cleaning. Most of this was carried out by the ward domestic, assisted by the cleaner, who worked under her. One of the jobs was to wipe over all the patients' lockers with a mild disinfectant solution twice a day. In the morning this was usually done by the cleaner, but on her days off and in the evenings the job generally fell to me as the junior. It was something I never minded doing since it gave me a chance to talk to patients as I tidied up around them and was able to make sure they had everything they needed within reach before moving on to the next bed. The thing that nobody looked forward to, however, was 'Cleaning Morning'.

Cleaning Morning happened once a week on the medical wards. The ward was done half at a time, so that it was all thoroughly cleaned once a fortnight. We started by moving all the beds from one side out to the middle of the ward, so that the bottom of the bed was nearly to the bottom of the one opposite. Then we started cleaning the side that had been cleared, with the cleaners concentrating on doing the floor. The first couple of times I waited to be told what to do and as a result I got the worst job, cleaning the wheels of all beds and lockers. This involved not just washing them but scraping away any dirt with an old knife kept for the purpose. After that I became cannier and on the next occasion announced that I thought I should do the high dusting as I was tall and could reach more easily than the others. At the same time, before anyone could argue, I grabbed the pole with duster attached that was specially designed for this purpose. From then on this was my job, dusting all the rails around the beds, plus high ledges and windows and finally helping to change the curtains.

Cleaning morning was a particular feature of the medical wards. On the surgical wards not only did nurses have too much else to do, but it would be impossible to pull all the beds out from one side because there would always be patients being prepared for or having just come back from surgery. Their beds would need to stay at the side so that curtains could be drawn around. Most other wards had smaller rooms which were cleaned entirely by domestic staff. Since all wards had their own domestics and cleaners, they were part of the ward team and took a keen pride in their work, something often sadly missing when such work is contracted out as it is today.

Moving beds out to the middle of the ward could sometimes cause problems however. Occasionally, if someone was particularly unwell we just had to leave them where they were and miss cleaning that area that week. One week when we were well into the cleaning there was suddenly a dreadful noise, a load rasping gasp from one of the patients who was lying on her bed in the middle of the ward. Everybody looked up. Kay and I were both close by and after glancing at each other, simultaneously we dropped what we were doing, quickly pulled the bed back to the side and drew the curtains around. The woman was unconscious and pulseless. A doctor was called and he attempted cardiac massage, but to no avail. She had had a massive heart attack and died instantly. Apart from cardiac massage, little more was done in an attempt to resuscitate patients then. There were no such things as crash calls, and as far as I knew only the operating theatre had a defibrillator. I certainly never saw it used in all my time training.

This was a shock to all of us, including most of the other patients, who must have been aware of what had happened. But no one said anything much. We just quietly got on with our work.

7.

Gaining experience

It was inevitable that there would be times when we were upset by the things we witnessed, and of course this worried me at first. But there was no way these things could be avoided and I never wanted to give up because of anything I saw. I told myself that if I was not there these things would still happen, so surely I should be able to face them, and after all it was far worse for patients and families involved. At least I could do my best to support them. Mostly, though, I was kept so busy that there was little time to dwell upon anything.

I soon began to understand a bit about the more common conditions that had brought the patients into the ward. Those coming in following a coronary thrombosis (heart attack) were initially given bed rest and started on digoxin and anticoagulant drugs to reduce the chances of further blood clotting in their narrowed coronary arteries. The doses of the anticoagulants had to be carefully monitored and daily blood samples were taken for checking clotting times, because if they had too high a dose, the blood clotted too slowly and there was the danger of bleeding. Their dose had to be stabilized before they went home. We could have hardly imagined the sort of treatments available today, where it is possible to use a catheter inserted via blood vessels leading to the heart so that a blood clot blocking a coronary artery may sometimes actually be removed and a stent, a small tube, inserted to keep the vessel open. Coronary bypass operations, where a healthy blood vessel is taken from somewhere else in the body and grafted onto the heart so that blood can bypass the constriction of the coronary artery to maintain blood supply to the heart muscle, had just been introduced in the US, but we had still never heard of it here.

We usually had two or three diabetics come in to stabilize their insulin dosage, plus some being admitted in a coma due to either too high or too low blood sugar levels, in which case they would first need treatment with either insulin or a glucose drip. Before meals they provided us with a urine sample to be tested for sugar, which you did by taking a fixed number of drops of urine and water in a test tube and adding a reagent in the form of a tablet. This fizzed up and, if sugar was present, the solution changed colour from blue (no sugar) through green and yellow to orange, according to the amount present. Depending on the result they were prescribed appropriate amounts of insulin. A second person always checked this out as the insulin solution could come in several different strengths and the amount given needed careful calculation. It is important that diabetes is controlled as well as possible because, if blood sugar levels are too high, over time it leads to severe complications such as blindness and nerve damage. However for sugar to be excreted in urine the blood sugar levels are already raised a bit above normal, so these slightly raised levels were not detected. Testing of blood sugar from finger pricks, which is more accurate, was being developed at this time and soon to be introduced, but then we still had to rely on urine testing.

Some of the most upsetting cases for me on the medical wards were those who had suffered strokes. There were, I learnt, two kinds of stroke. One, the most common, was where blood clots within a narrowed blood vessel causing it to become blocked. This cuts off the circulation to part of the brain, which leads to damage of the affected area. The effect of the stroke depends on which part of the brain is damaged. Because of the way the nervous system is structured, if the left side of the brain is damaged it affects the right side of the body, and vice versa. Mrs Arbuthnot was one such patient. Her left brain was damaged and the right side of her body was completely paralyzed. What is more, the left side of the brain includes the speech centre, so she was now unable to speak or write. Her mind was quite normal, but she was unable to express herself. The frustration this must cause is almost unimaginable.

Today when anyone has a stroke there are drugs that can be given to dissolve the clot and so restore circulation to the brain. If this is done fast enough the brain can often make a good recovery, or certainly better than it would otherwise. We didn't have such good drugs then, and the importance of rapid treatment was not realised. Therefore, although anticoagulants were given, most recovery depended on good nursing care and physiotherapy, a very long process. The outlook for Mrs Arbuthnot was not good. After a couple of weeks she was transferred to a nursing home for long term care. Whether she was ever able to go home I never knew.

Less commonly a stroke is really the opposite in that it is due to a haemorrhage. These strokes are due to a blood vessel rupturing and bleeding into the space around the brain, the subarachnoid space which separates the brain tissue from the skull. It is important to distinguish between the two types of stroke because it would be extremely dangerous to give anticoagulants to reduce blood clotting to someone who has had a bleed. Today the two can be readily distinguished by scans, but then the only way was by a lumber puncture. A small sample of the fluid that surrounds both the brain and spinal cord is taken, which can be done by inserting a needle between the vertebrae of the lower back, and then examining it for the presence of blood. If blood is present the cause of the stroke is a haemorrhage. At the same time the pressure of the fluid is measured by attaching a manometer, a long glass tube, to the needle. The tube is then held vertically and the fluid runs up, the extent of which depends on its pressure. The side of the tube is calibrated so that it can be measured accurately.

After I had been on the ward for a few weeks Mrs Benson was admitted following a stroke that had started with a sudden severe headache, signs that it could be a haemorrhage. She was to have a lumber puncture and Staff Nurse told me I was to assist, but first I had to prepare the trolley with all the necessary equipment for the doctor to use. Of course nothing was disposable then, so everything had to be sterilized.

All the instructions I needed were in the Procedure Book, of which there was a copy in every ward. This book, kept in Sister's office, contained detailed instructions for the correct way to carry out every possible procedure you were likely to come across as part of your duties as a nurse, so this is where I went to find out exactly what I needed to prepare the trolley.

Every ward had a sterilization room where all equipment for sterile procedures was to be found. There was a large water filled sterilizer, kept constantly near boiling point, which contained a variety of different sized bowls, kidney dishes and their lids. I first checked that there were enough containers and turned up the heat so that it would boil for at least five minutes. Then I moved to the small instrument sterilizer, which was on a bench at the side. Into this I placed the special lumbar puncture needle plus a spare and the glass manometer before turning this up to boil as well.

The trolley had first to be cleaned with spirit. Then, once the sterilizers had boiled for long enough, I turned them down again and used the long forceps that were kept standing in antiseptic solution to remove what I needed. The top was laid with the sterile equipment, bowls filled with swabs, another bowl for antiseptic solution and the

56

manometer plus needles in its own long metal container. The bottom shelf included packs containing sterile towels to drape over the patient and sterile surgical gloves for the doctor, as well as a bowl for rubbish. Staff Nurse got a bottle of local anaesthetic solution from the drugs cupboard and added it to the bottom. She then checked that I had everything I needed.

When the doctor arrived I brought the trolley to the bedside and helped Mrs Benson into the correct position. She had to be on her side with her back to the doctor and right to the edge of the bed, curled round as far as she could so as to separate her spinal vertebrae as much as possible. I then assisted the doctor by opening the packet of gloves so that he could put them on without touching the outside of the pack, then holding the bottle of local anaesthetic for him to withdraw some into the syringe. After that it was a matter of helping Mrs Benson keep still and in the right position, plus giving her words of encouragement, while the doctor got on with the procedure.

There was blood in the sample of fluid. That meant her stroke had been due to a bleed. As her blood pressure was rather high she was treated for this in hope that it would reduce the chances of a further bleed. If this had happened today she would have had a scan rather than lumbar puncture and from this it might be possible to determine the cause of the bleed, which could be due to an aneurysm, a swelling of one of the arteries in the brain. These slowly weaken over time and can eventually rupture, and need to be repaired surgically to prevent further bleeding. We didn't have facilities for neurosurgery at our hospital, the nearest centre for this being in Bristol. I don't remember if any further investigations or treatment were ever planned for Mrs Benson, but she seemed to recover well and was eventually discharged home.

Although the average age of patients was probably around seventy, there were some younger ones. These sadly were often overdoses. They would have had their stomachs washed out while in Casualty, where they would also have a drip set up and a catheter inserted if still unconscious, before being admitted to the ward. Once they had come round they would be seen by a psychiatrist before deciding whether they could go home or need further treatment at a psychiatric hospital. Some overdoses weren't serious attempts but more cries for help, considered by some to be attention seekers. Others were definitely serious attempts at taking their own lives. I found it hard to imagine how anyone could be driven to do this, but then I had come from a stable home background and who knows how I would have reacted in their circumstances. I always wished I could have talked to them more to try to understand, but I didn't really know what to say and as a junior it wasn't my job anyway. But some staff were not very sympathetic and to an extent I could see why. When you are looking after so many seriously ill people, ill through no fault of their own, some might feel their time was being taken up unnecessarily.

This attitude was exemplified by Joan Derby. She was a fellow student nurse in her first year who I only knew by sight. When she came in having taken an overdose of sleeping tablets she was admitted to the main ward rather than the side room normally reserved for staff. It was as if she was being punished for her action. Her attempt at her life had been a serious one. It turned out that she had a baby at home being looked after by her parents while she trained. This being the early sixties, having an illegitimate child was still considered rather shocking, at least by the older generation, although I think my generation was beginning to be a bit more liberal. Joan must have found the pressure too much and she never returned to her training.

With so many acutely ill patients it was inevitable that not all would survive and I would soon have to face the prospect of having someone die when I was on duty. I didn't have to wait long. Mrs Gutteridge was a sixty year old woman who had aplastic anaemia. In this condition the bone marrow fails so that it no longer produces blood cells. The most obvious first symptom is anaemia, but other blood cells involved in fighting infection and in clotting are also affected, so she was also prone to infections and to bruising. She had been in hospital for treatment before, when she had been given blood transfusions, but although she did have more blood given to her now, it only had a very temporary affect.

I was on duty with Staff Nurse Norland that evening. We had moved Mrs Gutteridge to a bed at the end of the ward near the entrance and her daughter was allowed to stay and sit with her with the curtains drawn around. Her husband had died some years ago so she had no other family. All other visitors had gone and we were attending to one of the other patients when were heard the daughter crying softly. Staff Nurse looked at me, and went quickly to Mrs Gutteridge's bedside. She had just died.

A doctor came to certify the death and shortly afterwards her daughter said her final goodbye and left the ward. Dealing with distressed relatives was, I came to discover, often the hardest part to handle when someone dies. Now we had to lay out her body.

'Are you alright with this?' Staff Nurse asked.

I nodded and steeled myself to join her behind the curtains. There was nothing really to worry about. Mrs Gutteridge looked at peace. Her colour, which had already been pale due to her anaemia in life, now had a bluish tinge. She was still slightly warm, but becoming cooler.

We gave her a final wash. We had to close her eyes and put a bandage around under her chin and over her head to keep her mouth shut. Finally we combed her hair, put her in a white shroud and attached a label with her name and details. Her belongings were put into a special bag and labelled. Her daughter would collect this from the administration office later. Then we called a porter, who arrived with the mortuary trolley. Before he came in we drew the curtains around all the other nearby patients so they wouldn't see what was happening, although I am sure most of them knew. We then helped the porter move Mrs Gutteridge across onto the trolley and he closed the large metal lid over her body so that it was completely hidden before taking her away down to the mortuary.

It is always sad to lose a patient that you have nursed and got to know. At the same time I was glad I had managed to cope with it alright for the first time. There would be more deaths to deal with in the future, although I don't think I ever had to lay out more than three or four more patients in the whole course of my training.

Aplastic anaemia is quite a rare condition. I believe today it can often be treated successfully by carrying out a bone marrow transplant.

I don't know what gave her the idea, but one day in the classroom Pat announced suddenly that she thought it would be good for us to see a post mortem (PM). It would complete our study of anatomy and physiology. The sister tutors were a bit taken back by the request but thought it should be possible, and they asked the rest of us what we thought. We all agreed rather cautiously. So Sister Underwood said she would have a word with the pathologist to see if he was agreeable to having us come to watch.

We were now having weekly study days and the following week when we arrived in the classroom we were told that it had all been arranged for later that morning.

'None of you have to do this if you don't want to,' Sister Underwood emphasised. 'It isn't part of the course so don't feel you are under any pressure. And if you do go, you can leave at any time.'

I admit I wasn't totally sure, but I had already seen an operation and laid out a body, so thought I should be able to cope. The others all seemed keen and I knew I would regret it if I missed the opportunity, as it might never arise again. So at the allotted time we all trouped rather nervously over to the hospital mortuary with Sister Underwood leading the way.

Today realistic scenes of mortuaries are probably depicted every week on television as part of detective dramas, to say nothing of every episode of series like 'Silent Witness'. It was not so then and I really didn't know quite what to expect. After putting on gowns we were led in to the PM room. There were two large slabs in the centre. One was being hosed down by a man who turned out to be the mortuary assistant and on the other slab lay the body of a grey haired woman. There were also two other men present, standing at the back of the room, one of whom was a young police officer.

The pathologist was there and ready to start. After greeting us he told us a bit about the background of the woman on whom he was to perform the post mortem. Apparently she had collapsed very suddenly when out shopping and was rushed to hospital by ambulance, only to be found dead on arrival. There were no reasons to think that she had died of anything other than natural causes, but the PM was needed to determine the exact cause of death and because it was a sudden death a police officer was present.

There were no external injuries, so the pathologist quickly got down to the real business.

'We always start at the head.' He explained. 'This is the bit that sometimes worries people most, so you may like to look away when I start with the saw.'

He then quickly peeled part of the scalp forward and removed the top of the skull with an electric saw. None of us looked too closely at this point. However after he had removed the brain over to the bench at the side to examine it, we began to look more interested and moved a bit closer to see this almost jelly like organ with its intricately convoluted surface. You could see very clearly the different areas of grey and white mater, the grey being the nerve cell bodies and the white being the long nerve processes. Looking at it I couldn't help being amazed that it is able to do so much, controlling movement, making us aware of sensations such as sight and sound and being the seat of our consciousness, enabling us to think and store knowledge. It gives us our personalities.

'This all looks perfectly normal and healthy,' said the pathologist as he examined the brain carefully. 'She did not die of a stroke.'

He replaced the brain and moved on to the body, making a large Y shaped incision and removing part of the chest wall. He then removed the different organs one by one, weighed and examined each of them thoroughly as he showed them to us. We looked at the heart and then the other organs in turn; the lungs, liver, kidney, spleen, gall bladder, intestines, uterus and ovaries.

When he looked at her heart he soon found the cause of death. It had been a heart attack. The coronary arteries that maintain the blood supply to the heart muscle had become completely blocked. Cutting off the blood supply meant that a large area of the heart muscle had been so severely damaged that it had just stopped beating.

Once finished all the organs were replaced back in the body. I was a bit surprised they weren't replaced in exactly the same position as in life, but I suppose it didn't matter. The assistant now took over and did the stitching up with large stitches, not like the neat ones I had seen in the operating theatre. While the PM had been going on the assistant had finished cleaning the other slab and there was now the body of a man laid out ready for the pathologist to move on to next.

Before we left the pathologist explained briefly about some of the forms he needed to fill in and send to the coroner, which all had to be done before the relatives could arrange her funeral. We returned to the classroom.

'Well, what did you think? Was it useful to you?' Sister Underwood asked.

'Fascinating!' Pat replied. 'You could really see things we have been taught, like the heart valves and the lobes of the liver and . . .so much.'

We all murmured our agreement.

'Good. Well you can now all go to off to lunch and I'll see you back in the classroom this afternoon.'

We trouped off.

'I hope it's not liver for lunch.' said Nancy.

8.

Night duty

We were all expected to do a minimum of three months night duty every year of our training, and it could be longer; over four months and even five were not unknown. The work rota was based on a fortnight rather than a week, during which we worked ten nights on and four off. That meant you could work anything up to twenty consecutive nights if you had your four nights off at the beginning of one fortnight and the end of the next. I never did this—I think the most I did was sixteen—but it did happen to others.

Before going on duty for our first night we all had to work the morning on the ward, which was somehow supposed to make up our hours, and this was useful as it gave us the chance to find our way around the new ward and get to know the patients a bit. Then, after lunch, we had to have all our belongings packed up as we were to move to new accommodation, specially reserved for those of us on nights. Our new rooms were in the wing of a nursing home on the other side of town where it was quiet and we wouldn't be disturbed when sleeping during the day. And it was quiet. All we could hear from there was the sound of the sea as waves broke on the cliffs below and the cry of gulls.

Hilary and I were to share a room and, after we had unpacked, we made some attempt to get some sleep before it was time to get ready for our first night on. We had transport provided in the form of a minibus to take us up to the hospital in the evenings in time to have supper and we would have breakfast there in the morning before being brought back. There was a small kitchen that we could use during the day to make hot drinks and toast if we needed. There were only three or four other students living there, as most became non-resident during their second year.

I was to work on Men's Medical. Having already worked on Women's Medical, at least I was familiar with most of their conditions. I was on with Staff Nurse Stevens, who worked permanently on nights. Coming on duty at 9.45 p.m. my first task was to start settling patients for the night while Staff Nurse did the medicine round, giving out sleeping pills. The work was rather easier than on the women's ward as there were no bedpan rounds. Instead I had to collect used bottles in a metal rack, which could be wheeled round the ward, and take these to the sluice. Once emptied and washed, the clean bottles had to be given out again and most of the men kept one for the night. Then there were patients who needed turning and pressure areas treated, which we did together, and four hourly observations of TPR and blood pressure to be recorded. Finally we went round making sure everyone was as comfortable as possible for the night. By 10.45 p.m. the lights were out.

We sat at the table in the centre of the ward with an angle poise lamp set up with a dark green cloth over to shield the beam from the patients, just focusing the light on anything we needed to read or write. When we had a patient who needed a lot of attention during the night we would also put cloth over their bedside light to make it less disturbing for the others when we had to turn it on.

At midnight Staff Nurse went to first dinner.

'If you have any problems Nurse Henderson is next door,' she said. Nurse Henderson was a third year student.

I was handed the keys and left alone. I wandered down the silent ward in the semi-darkness, checked a couple of drips to make sure they were running at the correct rate, then sat at the table and studied the Kardex to help me memorise the patients' names and what they were all in for.

It was all so different from during the day; everything quiet, just a few snores to reassure me that they were sleeping.

When Staff Nurse returned it was my turn for dinner. In the dining room I met up with Nancy, who was on Gynae.

'I'm not very hungry,' I said. 'It's not that long since supper.'

'Neither am I really, but we'd better have something,' she replied. 'It's a long time 'till breakfast. Do you think we'll ever manage to keep awake that long?'

I had been wondering the same thing. It was only 1 am, so we had another seven hours to go.

Back on the ward it was still all quiet. There were a couple of patients who needed turning regularly and Staff Nurse had to wake one or two others to give them their medication. Every so often one of us would walk around the ward to see if everyone was alright and check the drips. Apart from that we were able to sit down for much of the time, just getting up every so often if someone needed something, like their bottle emptying, or perhaps a drink. I made several cups of tea for those lying awake. It got quite cool when we were just sitting, but we were allowed to wear navy cardigans over our uniform and had our cloaks with us to wear when going to meals. While we were quiet Staff Nurse took time to explain to me more about what needed to be done.

'I know it's quiet now,' she said, 'but the morning is the really busy time, so you need to be well prepared. There will be the early morning teas, and you can get the trolley ready for that now. When we wake them in the morning there are the TPRs first, then teas and then washes. Those who can't do themselves it's just face and hands, and backs of course. That'll be Mr Timms, Mr Smales . . .' She indicated which patients would need help.

'Then there are the diabetics. You need wee samples from them for testing.' This would be urine samples that had to be tested for sugar. They would need their insulin before breakfast.

'—and all the bowls must be cleared up and everyone ready for breakfast by the time the day staff arrive. Then, while I am giving the report, you can help Mrs York start breakfasts. Oh, and there are the fluid charts. They must be fully completed before we go.' I knew about these. The fluid balance charts ran for 24 hours from 8 am to 8am the next day, so I would have to add up the final totals and put out new charts for the next 24 hours.

I looked at my watch. Still only 3am. I was beginning to feel really sleepy, but still a long time to go.

At 4 am it was tea time, Staff Nurse first and then me. Sitting down for tea I was really beginning to find it difficult to stay awake. I wondered how on earth I was going to have enough energy to cope with the morning rush! Hilary was there and she looked as bad as me.

Back on the ward Mr Timms was awake and wanted to sit up a bit.

'We can get him done now,' Staff Nurse said. 'If we give him his wash now, that'll be one less for later.' It was 5.30.

At 6 am Staff Nurse put the lights on, but kept them turned down to dim at first. Looking out of the window I could see the first glow of dawn. After that I had no more time to think of tiredness; it was one mad rush to get everything done. At last the day staff arrived and Staff Nurse disappeared with them into the office to give the report. I was still adding up the fluid balance charts and saw Mrs York, the ward domestic, arrive and go into the kitchen. Shortly afterwards she reappeared with the breakfast trolley. She made no comment to me, so the kitchen must have been tidied to her satisfaction.

I then started helping serve breakfast, giving out tea, cereal, boiled eggs and toast, until the day staff came out of the office and took over. I was off duty at last, and with relief made my way up to the dining room for my own breakfast.

Up in the dining room we tucked into our eggs and bacon with a feeling of euphoria, not uncommon after a night duty shift. Hilary was the last to join us.

'Gosh, what a night,' she sank thankfully onto her seat. 'We had three admissions!' She was on Men's Surgical.

'I heard that there'd been bad road accident brought into Casualty,' said Pat.

'Yes, two were from that—one quite a nasty head injury—and we had a bowel obstruction as well who had to go to theatre. It's been non-stop.'

'Nothing as exciting as that for me,' said Pat, 'just confused old ladies on Women's Medical. One kept calling out really loudly for Peter, waking up half the ward. I don't know who Peter is, but probably her husband who's been dead for years.'

'My patients slept all night,' said Nancy who was on Gynae. 'It was really difficult staying awake with nothing to do, but we may get busier tonight because it's operating day today.'

Back at our new accommodation Hilary and I got on well together sharing a room and we both slept soundly throughout the day, the room kept dark with extra thick curtains. Some days I would wake and feel hungry, usually at about the time I would normally have lunch. I would creep out of the room and make myself toast and a milky drink of hot chocolate or horlicks in the kitchen, sometimes meeting one of the others there. After that I would quickly get back to sleep.

The atmosphere on nights was completely different from days, so much more relaxed and informal. As the weeks passed I began to enjoy myself. Staff Nurse Stevens and Nurse Spinks, the third year student who took charge when

Staff Nurse had her nights off, were both easy to get on with. I quickly got used to the routine. Most nights were similar to the first, although could be busier when we had admissions or a very ill patient.

The main problem we encountered was the one Pat commented on after the first night; some patients, who were no more than perhaps mildly forgetful during the day, could get very confused, perhaps calling out for their husband or wife, who as often as not had died some years earlier. Waking up in the strange environment of the hospital didn't help. Others would try to get up out of bed thinking it was morning and it could take quite a time to settle them down again. It did, however, also lead to some amusing incidents.

One involved Mr Hopkins, who had a habit of getting up and wandering round the ward. One night we were behind the curtains attending to someone else when we heard an anguished yell from further down the ward. Mr Hopkins had got up while we weren't looking and, after walking round the ward, couldn't remember where his bed was, so he was getting into one that was already occupied! The poor occupant had been rudely awakened.

Another patient was Mr Drake, who used to be a sailor. He was often incontinent and we had tried him with a catheter, but he'd managed to pull it out, which must have been painful because there is a balloon blown up with water on the inside that normally prevents it falling out. So now we just put a bottle in place which, of course, often got dislodged. One night at around 3 am he began to make a noise, starting quietly.

'Whoa, whoa.' he went on, became louder, then—'it's leaking! The boats leaking! There's water! It's filling up!'

Staff Nurse and I looked at each other and started to giggle. We both knew what had happened. We went quickly to his bedside and tried to calm him down, but to little avail.

He was now shouting. Most of the ward was awake and those who had cottoned on to what was going on were beginning to laugh as well. We changed his sopping wet bed and gave him a wash, making him comfortable again. Eventually he settled. I then went round offering tea to the rest of the patients who were wide awake.

Some nights Mr Drake was much worse than this, becoming very noisy and aggressive, and on a couple of occasions had to be sedated. We didn't do this lightly, but with a ward full of patients trying to sleep, we felt we had no choice.

I believe this problem is becoming worse in hospitals today. With an aging population there are inevitably more people with dementia of one sort or another. Nurses have been accused of sedating disruptive patients so that they can have a quiet time themselves, but I find that hard to believe. More likely there are other patients to consider. From my own experience in hospital I know at first hand just how distressing it can be when you are feeling unwell and worried yourself, and you have another patient nearby, confused, noisy and shouting, and being generally disruptive.

During our last month on nights the next set joined us. Probably with us being such a small set they needed more juniors. They now moved to join us at the Headland. We were quite a crowd travelling to and from work in the minibus. In the mornings we would wait for our transport in the common room, all feeling tired. Our tiredness after a busy night often made us slightly hysterical, laughing at the slightest thing.

'Have you ever seen a dead person's knees?' I thought I heard Pat say one morning.

We all looked rather puzzled.

'One of our women did a couple of minutes after. I suppose sneezing is a reflex.'

In my tired mind I slowly realised what Pat had really said as one of the others spoke up.

'But what happened to her knees?'

'I said have you ever seen a dead person *sneeze,* not person's knees.'

We all roared with laughter.

I had enjoyed my time on nights, but eventually our three month stint came to an end. Back on days I was next allocated to Women's Surgical—and Sister Lamb.

9.

Dragons

Some people think that in the sixties all matrons and ward sisters were dragons, but in reality the vast majority were perfectly approachable and fair with staff. If anyone was reproached by them it was almost always deserved. However we had a couple who would definitely go into the 'dragon' category. One of these was one of the Assistant Matrons, Miss Vernon. Rumour had it that she started working there in the dim and distant past as a domestic. She went on to do her nurse training and had been there ever since, rising to her present position. She missed nothing. If you passed her in the corridor she would notice anything slightly out of order in your uniform; if your apron wasn't clean and fresh, your stocking seams not straight, or you hair wasn't clear of your collar—a frequent problem for me as I didn't like mine too short. The other was Sister Lamb, the sister in charge of Women's Surgical. Like Miss Vernon she was considered one of the 'old school' and both were not too far from retirement.

On my first morning on Women's Surgical I joined the rest of the staff in the office for the report from the night staff. Sister Lamb was there, a well built and imposing woman with iron grey hair. She said very little during the report and, when finished, sent everybody off to start work, but before I could follow she got up and looked at me hard.

'So, where have you been working so far?' she asked.

I told her which wards I had been on and that I had just finished nights. She gave a grunt and continued to scrutinize me, looking down her nose as if I was something the cat had brought in.

'Well, you had better get on with it,' she said finally, and I joined the others in the ward.

As well as a staff nurse there were two other students on with me that morning, Tess Cameron, a fairly new first year and Val Ross, in her second year. At 9 am Staff Nurse and Tess were sent to coffee, leaving me and Val to go round doing the backs. Although some of the patients were mobile, at least half of them needed their pressure areas treated, and before we realised it the others were back from coffee. Sister Lamb came out of the office.

'Haven't you finished that yet?' she demanded when she saw that we still had three or four patients to go. 'What have you been doing? You should have finished easily by now. Well, you will have to go to coffee anyway and the others can finish off.'

We both remained silent and left the ward.

'Don't worry about it' Val said to me as we made our way up to the dining room. 'Though really, there's no way we could get round all those patients in just 30 minute.'

This was true. With around fifteen patients to treat in just half an hour that would be only two minutes each, impossible if we did the job properly plus washed our hands between each patient. But there was no point in arguing so we just had to ignore it.

Mornings were always the busiest time. As well as the routine bedpans and backs there were drips that had to be checked regularly and observations that needed doing as often as every 15 minutes on some patients. One of us juniors would usually be given the specific responsibility for these observations. They might include pulse and blood pressure on patients following surgery, or testing pupil reactions and state of consciousness on anyone following a head injury. Pupil reactions were tested by flashing a light into each eye separately and you had to note not just that they reacted but whether or not they were equal. Any changes might be the first signs of serious complications such as bleeding beneath the skull causing pressure on the brain.

This routine work was punctuated by admissions, either routine for surgery the next day, or emergencies, such as people with appendicitis, bowel obstructions, head injuries and broken bones that needed pinning, to name but a few. A staff nurse usually organized the operating lists, seeing that patients were given their premeds at the appropriate time. We would have to prepare patients and go with them to theatre when the porter arrived to collect them. Either a staff nurse or senior student did the dressings and removed any drains, stitches or clips that needed doing. Patients stayed in until they had all these removed, usually six days after their operation.

Mrs Bainbridge was one of the first patients I admitted there. She had come in with severe abdominal pain and what is known as 'faecal' vomiting, which, as its name implies, is dark brown and unpleasant smelling, signs of a bowel obstruction. The reason this happens is that some material in the gut above the obstruction can be regurgitated back into the stomach, from where it is vomited—not at all pleasant.

The doctor put up a drip and I was given the task of inserting a naso-gastric tube, known as a Ryle's tube. It was the first time I had carried out this procedure, but we had been taught how to do it at PTS, so I was pleased to get the experience. The tube is inserted via a nostril down the patient's throat and into their stomach. It is then used to aspirate the stomach contents, keeping it empty and so preventing further vomiting. After collecting everything I needed I explained to Mrs Bainbridge what I was going to do and why. First I measured the tube against her to estimate the length needed for it to reach her stomach. Then I lubricated the end of the tube and inserted it into a nostril. It went in easily and I pushed it gently into her throat. Next was the tricky bit. I had to make sure the tube went into her oesophagus, which leads to the stomach, and not into her lungs. Also the presence of a tube in the throat often makes people gag and the end of the tube can then come out of the patient's mouth. I told her to swallow and as she did I pushed the tube further, before pausing. I repeated this process a couple more times, until I judged that it should have reached her stomach. I then attached a large syringe to the tube and aspirated some fluid. This I tested with litmus paper, which showed it was acid, a clear sign that it was in the stomach. Finally I taped the tube to her face so that it stayed in position.

I was pleased with myself at having accomplished this successfully. Staff Nurse checked it was all correct—Sister Lamb was off duty that day—and said it was fine. Over the next few weeks I had more practice on other patients, soon becoming proficient in the procedure.

In the meantime Mrs Bainbridge was taken to theatre to find the cause of and relieve the obstruction. There are a number of possible causes of bowel obstruction, one of which is cancer. Luckily in her case it turned out to be due to diverticulitis, where part of the large intestine (gut) is inflamed. Over time scarring occurs which constricts, leading to a blockage. The affected section of her gut was removed and the ends sewn back together and she had to be given a temporary colostomy to give her gut time to heal. The colostomy bag needed changing regularly and Val showed me how it was done and how to treat the skin around, which can become quite sore where the bag is stuck to it. Once she was up and about she learnt to do this herself ready to go home. She would have to come back at a later date for the colostomy to be closed and get her back to normal.

It isn't pleasant having surgery at the best of times, but it was often much harder for the patients then than it is today. One example was the treatment of breast cancer.

Mrs Jarvis was a sixty year old lady who had found a lump in her breast, which could be cancer, but might be simply a cyst. It wasn't possible to tell which it was without having it removed and examined directly. So she was taken to theatre and the lump removed. From there it was sent straight to the Path Lab, where their staff were ready waiting. They then did what was called a frozen section, which is basically freezing the sample and cutting an extremely thin slice from it to examine under the microscope to see if there are cancerous cells present. Everyone in theatre waited for the result, with the patient still anaesthetized. If the result was negative, everything would be fine. She would have her wound closed and be sent back to the ward to recover. If it was cancer she would have a radical mastectomy, where as well as the breast, the muscle beneath it and the glands from under her arm would all be removed.

This was the standard procedure. The idea was that a patient wouldn't have to undergo two operations with two anaesthetics. But what this boiled down to was that when Mrs Jarvis went to theatre she didn't know whether she was going to have a mastectomy or not. It must have been terrible for her.

Unfortunately for Mrs Jarvis it was cancer, and she had a radical mastectomy.

Today she would first have had a mammogram and a biopsy to make the diagnosis. She would then know exactly what she was going to have done. If cancer is in the early stages sometimes just removing the lump and some surrounding tissue is enough. In others a mastectomy is necessary, but the under arm glands can be biopsied and, if clear, can be left, which avoids later possible complications.

If the glands have all been removed, lymphatic drainage is affected and this can lead to lymphodoema, where the arm becomes swollen with fluid and extremely uncomfortable.

Another big advance today has been the introduction of breast care nurses. These nurses give support and information throughout treatment for cancer, as well as being involved is some of the treatment. Nurses play similar roles in other types of cancer as well and it is a good example of an area where nurses today have really been able to extend their role.

It was less than a couple of weeks until Christmas when I started on the ward. We all looked forward to it, especially those of us for whom it would be our first Christmas working there, even though it would mean we were separated from our families. The hospital held a special Christmas dinner for students the week before, where we were served by some of the ward sisters. It was the traditional meal of roast turkey and all the trimmings followed by Christmas pudding. Luckily I was off duty, so could go along with Hilary, and some other first years from the set after us. We all enjoyed ourselves. When I was eating the Christmas pudding I suddenly found myself biting on something hard. For a moment I thought I had broken a tooth, then I realised I had the sixpence!

On Christmas Eve we spent every spare moment putting up the decorations, which were delivered to the ward in several boxes in which they had been stored from last year. We had a large tree placed at the end of the ward to decorate as well. The ward looked really festive by the time we finished. In the evening there was Carol singing. As many as possible of us were expected to join in, so those of us finishing at 8 pm all went. We all had to wear our cloaks worn inside out so the red lining showed, and carried candles as we processed round all the wards with the lights dimmed. Some of the patients joined in the singing with us and everyone had a good time.

On Christmas day itself everyone was on duty all day; no one was allowed a day off. The general rule was that students could not have more than one Christmas off during their three years, and this could only happen if you booked holiday or were on nights, where the usual rota continued and some lucky people had nights off. During the morning Sister Lamb made sure none of us were slacking and everything was done as usual. At least having everybody on duty meant we were able to get all the routine work done without such a rush, especially as there were slightly fewer patients than usual. There was no routine surgery that week and as many patients as possible had been sent home, so we had more time for those remaining and getting them ready for their Christmas lunch. Some were able to get up to the table and those staying in bed had their trays decorated with tinsel and holly. On our ward one of the consultants came to carve the turkey. Everybody had a Christmas cracker and soon most patients were wearing their paper hats. Everybody seemed to be enjoying themselves. Even Sister Lamb seemed in a good mood.

In the afternoon when the visitors arrived and there was nothing much for us to do, we were allowed to take turns to have some time off to go and visit other wards to see their decorations. Tess and I were sent off together. First we went next door to Men's Surgical. The staff looked as though they were having more fun than us, with half of them crowded in the office eating chocolates from an enormous box. They offered us some and we took a couple each, even though we had already had some on our own ward.

'I must go to ENT,' said Tess. 'That's where Kathy's working.' So that is where we went next. Tess and her friend

Kathy Meadows had come together from Scotland to train here.

On ENT I met Kathy, a pretty girl with her blonde hair cut in a neat bob. We admired the decorations and were offered more chocolates. Many wards saved up boxes of chocolates given to them from grateful patients over the year so that they had them for Christmas, with the result that we had a large surfeit.

'What made you both choose to come here to train?' I asked Kathy and Tess.

'We wanted to come to England, but not to be in a big city and we wanted to be near the sea,' said Kathy. 'We live near the sea at home and I would miss it terribly if it wasn't nearby. You can hear the waves from our house.'

'You'll enjoy night duty then,' I said, and told them about the night staff's accommodation at the Headland.

Next we went to the children's ward where Hilary was working. She was busy clearing up after a child had been sick all over the floor. When she finished she came over to us.

She said 'That's the third one that's been sick. They are all far too excited and their parents have been bringing them in sweets—which they are not supposed to do—but it's difficult to stop them with it being Christmas. Would you like some chocolates?'

Returning to the ward and, with visiting over for the afternoon, it was back to the routine of more bedpans and backs. Thankfully Sister sent most of us off at 8 pm, with just herself, one of the Staff Nurses and a student, who actually volunteered, staying on until 10 pm. Although at the time some of us did feel we missed out a bit with the festivities on our ward, Sister Lamb was right to see that we put the patients first. After all it was their Christmas.

I had more Christmas fare a couple of days later when I went home for my days off. My parents had postponed their

Christmas dinner so that I could join them, together with my younger sister. So I did well that year.

10.

Struggling on

Christmas was over, and a new year began. That meant we had completed our first year of training. All of us in our set had passed our first year hospital exams and we were now looking forward to having our grey belts, which would show that we were no longer juniors. The year of training which you were in was designated by the colour of your belt. For the first year you had no belt, then a grey one in the second, and maroon in the third. When you passed your hospital final exams at the end of the third year you were awarded a black belt. You kept the black belt as a Staff Nurse, but only had your blue dress after you passed the State Finals.

Although I was looking forward to receiving my grey belt, I was determined not to let it go to my head. I remembered how I had met Julie, a first year student who had started on Women's Medical just before I had been moved on from there. She looked a bit fed up.

'What's the matter? ' I asked.

'Oh just work,' she replied gloomily.

'I thought you were enjoying it. You seemed happy enough when I was there, but don't you like it anymore?'

'Oh, yes,' she replied. 'The ward's great. It's just Nurse Partridge.'

I was surprised. Gillian Partridge was a couple of sets ahead of me, so I didn't really know her.

'She's just so bossy, always ordering us around as if she's in charge,' Sheila told me. 'Mind you I haven't made myself very popular with her.' She grinned. 'When she first started there she had the nerve to get us all together with her in the sluice, that's me and another first year. She said "There's two

81

juniors today and we need to get organized." She still hadn't got her grey belt then, so I looked around all innocent and said "No there's three juniors." She looked furious.'

I laughed, but it wasn't really funny. Gillian was making herself unpopular behaving that way—a big mistake. Happily it was something I never encountered, as I always found the more senior students friendly and helpful. I hope I was the same with those junior to me. It was as though we were all in it together and should help each other out.

Eventually we received our summons to Matron's office to be presented with our belts. We went in one by one and Matron said something about us living up to our new positions. Afterwards we all put them on and admired one another. Back on the ward Staff Nurse was the only on to comment, congratulating me. I went back to doing the bedpan round.

There was less than two weeks to go to our Preliminary State Exam, always known as Prelims, but I had developed a sore throat and was beginning to feel very unwell. I went to see Sister Edwards, the Home Sister, who took my temperature. It was over 100°F (we still used Fahrenheit then).

'Up you go to bed,' she said. 'I'll tell the ward.'

The doctor came to see me the next morning and confirmed I had flu. Sister Edwards came up to my room and took my temperature every four hours. In the evenings when she was off duty, this was done by whichever of the Assistant Matrons was on when they came over to the Nurses' Home. I was not allowed any visitors, although Hilary did pop her head round the door a couple of times when she was sure nobody was looking.

Meals were brought in to me from the hospital on a tray, but I felt awful and could hardly eat anything. After a few days to my amazement one evening I had a tap on my door and Matron herself came in. I sat up straight in bed, not feeling I should be lying down in her presence.

'Don't get up,' she said. 'How are you feeling? Any better?'

I said I was a bit better.

She looked at my supper tray. 'You've hardly eaten anything.'

'I'm just not hungry, but I did manage all the pudding.' I had hardly touched the main course, but thought I had done quite well to eat all the banana in custard.

'You need something lighter,' she said. 'What about scrambled eggs?'

I nodded. 'Yes, that would be nice.'

So the next day my diet changed and lighter food, more suitable for an invalid, arrived.

After about a week I was getting better, but was overdue to ring my parents. I hadn't been able to let them know I was ill or when I was next likely to get home. The phone booth was downstairs, so in the evening I went down to make my call. I had only just started to speak to my mother, saying I had flu, when Miss Vernon, the Assistant Matron, appeared suddenly.

'What are you doing?' she demanded. 'You shouldn't be here. You must stay in your room.'

I said that I was ringing my parents, but she still insisted that I went straight back to my room. I quickly told my mother that I had to go, put the phone down and did as I was told. I felt like a naughty child. Luckily my mother had the sense to ring Home Sister the next morning to find out how I was.

Although I was beginning to feel better I was concerned about my exam, only a few days ahead, and said this to Sister Edwards.

'Don't worry,' she said. 'I'll get the doctor to sign you off until Wednesday, so you can have a couple of days or so at home to recover before you come back to take the exams. You can start back at work after that.'

So I was able to go home for the next few days to recuperate. My parents came to pick me up and my mother, always thoughtful, brought some flowers for Sister Edwards to thank her for looking after me.

The day of the exams finally arrived. We had two three hour papers, one on anatomy and physiology and the other covering nursing and nutrition, both taken on the same day, which wasn't ideal. I was fine for the first paper, but by the afternoon I'd developed a dreadful headache and found the second one a real struggle. In the end I didn't complete all the questions required and knew I'd done badly. But at least it was over and, although I felt more like going to bed, we all went out for the evening to celebrate.

Back on the ward Sister Lamb continued to appear just when you least expected to check up on what you were doing. One day I had been told to give an enema to one of the patients, a procedure I was already used to carrying out. I got the woman to lie on her side, as we had been taught, inserted the rectal catheter and poured in the warm soapy fluid. The commode was ready beside the bed for her to use afterwards. Sister Lamb looked in.

'Why have you got her on her side?' she wanted to know.

'That's the way we've been taught,' I replied, a bit confused.

'Well it's much better to have her standing up and leaning over the bed. Then she can get straight on the commode after.'

A week or so later I had another enema to give, so this time gave it to the patient with her standing up. Once again Sister Lamb looked in.

'Why is she standing up?' she asked. 'You know the correct procedure is to have her on her side.'

What could I say?

I bit later I was told to prepare for a patient to have a lumbar puncture. It was quite unusual for this procedure to be carried out on a surgical ward, but I had prepared and assisted several times while on Women's Medical, so knew exactly what to do. I had to go to the medical ward to borrow the needles and monometer, and, after sterilizing everything, soon had the trolley ready. Sister Lamb came into the sterilization room. She looked around the room and at the trolley.

Where's the Procedure Book?' she demanded. 'You won't know everything you need if you don't follow the Procedure Book.'

'It's alright, I've got everything,' I replied. 'I've done this several times before on the medical wards.'

She looked at me disbelievingly and disappeared to collect the Procedure Book from her office. After consulting it, she scrutinized my work. I began to feel worried in case I had missed something, but she made no further comment, so must have been satisfied. No comment was probably the nearest she came to praise. After that she didn't check up on me so often and left me to get on with my work. It was as though it took a while before she fully trusted you to work on her ward with her patients.

Not everyone coped well with the pressure on Women's Surgical though, and I was glad it hadn't been my first ward. Tess had managed well, but by now she had moved on elsewhere and we had a new first year student fresh from PTS. This was Dawn Melrose, always anxious looking and terrified of Sister Lamb. When Sister did her usual trick of appearing suddenly to check up on what she was doing, poor

Dawn was all fingers and thumbs and couldn't do anything right.

'I knew it would be hard work,' she said to me during one lunch break, 'but it's different, so much harder than I thought. It's not just the work, but some of the cases we get. How can you go on after seeing some of the things you do?'

Of course there were times for all of us when we were upset by some of the things we saw, I told her, but it was part of the job and we couldn't let it affect our work. There never seemed time to dwell on things very much. But there had been one recent case on this ward that had upset us all. Mrs Henderson, still only in her twenties and not long married, came in with a large lump in her breast which was found to be cancerous. Sadly the disease had already spread to her lymph glands and lungs, so it was too far advanced for surgery and there was nothing that could be done.

"Why on earth didn't she do something about it sooner? Surely she noticed the lump,' Dawn asked when we were in the office together with Staff Nurse.

Staff Nurse shrugged. 'She mightn't have noticed it if she didn't examine herself often enough, or maybe she just hoped it would go away. Plus she would have had to wait several weeks for her appointment to be seen, so it could have grown in that time.'

That was true. Waits for outpatient's appointment were very much longer then, even for those with suspected cancer. Mrs Henderson was sent home with the prospect of radiotherapy to slow down the progress of the disease. Some people, like Dawn, just couldn't cope with this sort of thing, and after working her notice she left.

But Dawn wasn't the only one feeling depressed by it all. This was the time during my training when I felt at my lowest ebb, not so uncommon when students reach their second year, and made worse because I had to retake the exam that I had messed up after being ill. Also, although we were being given increasing responsibility, most of the time I still just carried on with the basic duties. I often felt strongly that I was supposed to be a student and I wasn't learning anything—and there was still such a long way to go.

I did seriously think about giving up. After all I had already lasted much longer than I had originally expected, but the trouble was I still hadn't thought of anything else I wanted to do—to say nothing of having to start at the bottom again with something else. Plus it seemed so defeatist. So I carried on with the endless bedpan and back rounds while feeling thoroughly fed up with it all. At the same time I did feel guilty at my thoughts; after all this basic care is so important to patients. I hope I always managed to hide such feelings from them.

Perhaps some of this was an after effect of flu; it was heavy work on the ward and I was certainly feeling tired much of the time. However by now I had worked there for twelve weeks and was due for a move, only I was still not on the change list. I vowed that if I wasn't moved by the end of the month I would go to Matron to say that I had to have a change. But I needn't have worried. A couple of weeks later my name was on the list.

11.

Children

The Children's ward was somewhere I had really been looking forward to working, so was pleased when I was allocated there. It was a large open ward, like most of the others, but with six cubicles partitioned off, three on each side near the entrance. These were used mainly for babies, and large windows to the cubicles allowed us to keep an eye on the occupants. The ward was brightened up with picture of animals and scenes from nursery rhymes adorning the walls. At the far end there was a day room for those able to get up to play and where parents could sit with their children during visiting.

Sister Atkins had only just taken over following the previous sister's retirement, but she had been a staff nurse there for several years, so knew the ward well. She was, I soon discovered, an avid supporter of the local football team and her weekends off were often timed to coincide with important matches. She clearly adored the children and was always so kind and gentle with them, helping to allay their fears on what must have been such a frightening experience for them at their age.

There was always a lot to do. There were the usual washes and baths and routine observations of TPRs and blood pressures. At mealtimes there were toddlers to feed and bottles for babies—one of the few times we could sit down. Drug rounds in particular could be hard work, with some children needing quite a bit of persuasion before they would swallow their medicine. I never enjoyed giving them injections. Some made a lot of fuss once they realised what was to happen and I could sympathize as I remembered how

I myself had been terrified of needles as a child. Newcomers were usually very quiet at first and we tried to spend a bit more time with them, but other children, who had been there a while and were up and about, were always good at going to talk to them and getting them involved. Within a day or two they would be talking and laughing with the rest.

I had often been impressed by the stoicism displayed by patients in the face their illness and treatment. Many children were the same, but they could show their distress in different ways. One example was Janet, a six year old who had broken her leg. It was her femur (thigh bone) and her leg needed to be in traction for around six weeks. This was a much shorter time than for an adult, who would have needed nearer twelve weeks in traction, but luckily children's' bones heal much faster.

Janet was a bright and cheerful little girl, often bouncing up and down on her bed once she got used to the traction. But she wet her bed.

'She's been dry for years, since she was two,' her mother told us. 'Janet love, you must say to one of the nurses when you want the toilet.'

Janet looked solemn but didn't say anything.

'It's just the upset with all she's been through,' Sister told her mother. 'She may settle down in time. We are going to try sitting her on a pan every two hours. We mustn't make a big deal about it or it will upset her more.'

But although we tried giving her bedpans more frequently, she often ended up with a wet bed, we would just find her already soaking wet when we brought it to her. If we sat her on a bedpan she would only sometimes use it, although would never ask for one herself when she needed it. But she never seemed worried about it and continued to be her usual cheerful self.

Eventually her six weeks were up and the traction removed. At first she was terrified to move, she had become so used to being on traction, but once she was on her feet she was able to go home. We hoped there would now be no more wet beds, but I never heard.

Visiting hours on the children's ward were the same as for adults. At this time some hospitals were beginning to have more open visiting for children and apparently it had been tried, but the previous ward sister hadn't liked it. She found it disruptive to the routine and children were easier to manage without parents there all the time. Not so many years before there had been no visiting allowed at all for children and I expect that was what she had been used to. The idea of getting parents involved in their children's care and treatment was foreign to many nurses then. Of course children did often cry and make a fuss when their parents left, but that is a quite normal reaction and it would have been more worrying if they didn't. But not all children had parents able to visit.

Mandy was a five year old whose mother, a single parent, had developed TB and was currently undergoing treatment in the chest hospital some distance away. Luckily Mandy hadn't caught the disease, but was not allowed any contact with her mother because of the infection. She had been looked after by foster parents for a while, but shortly after had developed rheumatic fever and been admitted to hospital.

Rheumatic fever can occur following on from a throat infection when it is caused by a particular bacteria, a strain of streptococci. The main problem is that it causes inflammation of the lining to the heart and this can lead to permanent damage to the heart valves if not treated. To avoid heart damage the treatment includes strict bed rest for three to four weeks, following which gentle activity can be started. By the time I started on the ward Mandy had already been there for a while and was now allowed out of bed to sit in a chair for a short time each day.

Needless to say Mandy missed her mother terribly and frequently became extremely upset, angry at first, followed by copious tears. One day Sister came into the ward and told me to get Mandy into a wheel chair quickly and bring her to the office. She had Mandy's mother on the phone. The delight on Mandy's face was amazing as I wheeled her to the office and she talked happily for a few minutes. Afterwards was the first time I saw her laugh, although followed by a few tears as I took her back to bed.

I think this really showed the importance of contact between children and parents. Just talking on the phone seems nothing special today with everyone having mobiles, but it was quite a big deal then. Patients were not normally allowed to use the hospital phones. For them there was a pay phone on a trolley that could be brought to the bedside and plugged in, and they often had to wait a while for this to be available. It was rarely used in the children's ward—children weren't expected to make phone calls. How times change!

Although Mandy was happier for a while, her tantrums soon returned. One day she became particularly upset.

'I'm going to my mum,' she shouted suddenly and ran out of the ward and away down the corridor. I went tearing after her and soon caught up. She collapsed on the ground sobbing and I just knelt down with her trying to give some comfort. When she was calm again we returned to the ward. Not long after this she was well enough to be discharged, to foster parents again until her own mother recovered. I don't know how long it was before she was able to be reunited with her mother.

There were, inevitably, a few tragic cases. One was Paul, a ten year old with leukaemia, always so polite and well behaved. He had been in and out of the ward several times before, but now he was deteriorating fast. I hadn't known him previously, but the permanent ward staff had all become really attached to him and were visibly upset. I went home for my days off and when I returned found he had died. I was just relieved that I hadn't been there at the time. Today childhood leukaemia can often be treated successfully with a bone marrow transplant, not heard of then.

Another was Michael, a six month old baby with meningitis. It was touch and go as to whether he would survive. His anxious parents sat quietly with him throughout every visiting hour. His breathing was shallow and we had to watch him carefully in case he stopped altogether. But he did survive. As he recovered he was first fed by a tube, but as he became stronger he began to take a bottle again. Even so his body felt limp and he wasn't as active as a baby of his age should be. Eventually he was able to go home with his thankful parents. But Sister did not look happy.

'I sometimes wonder what we are saving,' she said after they had gone. 'His long term prospects are not good, I'm afraid. He's sure to have some permanent brain damage, we just can't tell at this stage how much he will be affected.'

'Do his parents know?' I asked.

'They have been warned, but I don't think it's really sunk in. The trouble is we can't say just how he will be affected yet, so we don't like to be too pessimistic. So they are not really accepting it. Perhaps it's better that way, just finding out gradually.'

Of course we always had to appear cheerful in front of the children however we might feel, and there always seemed a happy atmosphere in the ward. The vast majority of the children underwent successful treatment and were discharged home happily. There was Peter with appendicitis, home a week later once he had his stitches out. Then Sally, one of the most angelic two year olds I have known with her blond hair. She had an operation to correct a squint. It is important that squints are corrected as early as possible. If they are done later than about the age of two, the vision in the so called lazy eye never catches up with the other.

Another boy we had in was three year old Matthew. Small children always like to put things in their mouths whenever possible, and the trouble with this is that the object is then sometimes swallowed. Coins are often ingested this way, although they usually get passed through the system without any trouble. However Matthew had swallowed an open nappy pin, and hence was admitted to the ward. The treatment for this was to give him a cotton wool sandwich, the idea being that the cotton wool would protect his gut as the pin passed through. I had the job of getting him to eat one.

I prepared the sandwich with sliced bread and put in plenty of butter and the jam over the layer of cotton wool, then cut it into small pieces to try to make it look a bit more appetizing. Getting him to eat it proved to be quite a challenge—he may not have been hungry anyway. However bit by bit he managed to get most of it down. By the end he was becoming really upset and Sister, who came to see how I was getting on, said he had had enough. So with relief I tucked him up in bed, telling him how good he had been. The pin was eventually passed successfully, and thankfully I didn't have the job of looking for it.

Although, as I have said, children new to the ward could be very quiet, after a while some could become quite boisterous and needed calming down.

Stephen was a seven year old who had broken his arm. It was a bad fracture involving his elbow, which always makes it difficult. He had been to theatre to have it set and put in plaster and now, the following day, he was allowed up. He made his way to the playroom to join a couple of the others. After a while it was getting quite noisy in there, with shouting and laughing and I glanced in, just in time to see Stephen, who was running at top speed round the room, slip and fall. He jumped up quickly.

'Are you alright?' I asked.

He nodded, but a minute later he made his own way back to bed looking subdued.

I told Sister what I had seen.

'Oh dear,' she said. 'I had better let the doctor know. In the meantime that will have to go on an accident form.'

An accident form had to be filled in for any incident such as this and would go to Matron's office. She would deal with anyone who might be responsible and, if necessary, review procedures to avoid such events happening again. She also kept a record in case there was any come back.

Stephen had to have his arm re-X-rayed, which showed the bone fragments had been dislodged once again. So now he was confined to bed with his arm suspended in traction to keep the broken bones aligned.

'What on earth did you think you were doing, running round like that, you silly boy,' his mother told him after Sister had explained to her apologetically what had happened. 'It's all your own fault. Now you will have to stay in bed.'

She blamed her son entirely. If that had been today the hospital would probably have been sued.

12.

Moving on

My next allocation was the Infection Ward. This ward was made up of around a dozen single rooms where patients could be nursed separately if they developed such things as wound infections after surgery or were having limb amputations because of gangrene. As well as this there was also the terminal care of some cancer patients. I didn't altogether like the sound of it at first, but in many ways my time there was a turning point for me. Sister Nash was one of the younger sisters and, with her lively sense of humour, she helped to create an excellent working atmosphere. As well as that Nancy was already working there. It was quite unusual for two people in the same set to work on a ward together and it was the only time it happened to me.

By now we were well into our second year and beginning to be given more responsibility. This including being able to do drug rounds on our own, although we still had to have certain categories of drugs checked out. There was only one Staff Nurse, so when either she or Sister had days off, Nancy and I would be left on together for either the afternoon or evening. Later, after Nancy had been moved on to her next ward, I would be on with a first year student.

Mr Warden was one patient we cared for. He had advanced cancer and was dying. When he had come in for surgery a short while ago it had revealed an inoperable cancer. Because of the cancer his wound never healed properly and continued to ooze a dark, blood stained liquid. He was now little more than a skeleton with no strength left. He had no family of his own having never married, just a sister who could only visit occasionally because she lived some distance away. He barely spoke as he laid there, waiting—and wanting—to die.

He was written up for morphine every four hours as needed, and had last been given a dose around lunch time. It was now 6 pm and I thought overdue for another dose. The assistant matron on for that evening came to do her rounds and see if there were any drugs that needed checking. I put out Mr Wardens chart for her.

'Does he need this?' she asked me.

'Yes, he had his last dose nearly six hours ago,' I replied.

'Let me see him.' This was a reasonable request and I showed her to his room.

'Hello Mr Warden,' she said. 'How are you? Are you in any pain?'

He said nothing, but looked at her and then slowly moved his head from side to side despairingly.

'Good.' She left the room, then to me. 'He doesn't need anything. He's not in pain.'

'But . . .' I stopped. I couldn't argue with an assistant matron. What I wanted to say was that he might not be in physical pain, although it was quite surprising that he wasn't, but what about his mental pain?

She went on. 'He is very weak. You know morphine can depress respiration?'

I nodded. This is well known.

'In his condition giving drugs like these could be enough to kill him.'

But he is dying anyway, I wanted to say. Did it matter if it was a bit sooner? It would be a happy release for him. This is a dilemma often encountered. Could you be bringing forward a patient's death by giving strong pain killers? Of course you wouldn't give them deliberately to cause death, but surely they shouldn't be withheld if they are needed and that is the most humane thing to do. But many nurses then seemed to be afraid to give them under these circumstances, even though they were written up by the doctor, who had obviously decided that the drugs were necessary. Sometime when I was in a less charitable mood I even wondered if they just didn't want a death while they were on duty.

Although many of the patients were seriously ill and in some cases dying, I found my work on the ward highly satisfying. I learnt a lot, had plenty of experience doing dressings and drug rounds and enjoyed being given more responsibility. So I felt things were generally looking up for me and this feeling was boosted further by moving out of the nurses' home. I had come to find the view out to the hedge rather depressing , especially as I would have liked to be able to see what was going on beyond, where the 'New Hospital' was beginning to take shape. Now I had a room in a house shared with Kay, who I had worked with on Women's Medical during my first year, plus a couple of others. Yet another factor was that we were now well into our second year study days, which were followed by a couple of weeks in study block.

This year we studied medicine, surgery, paediatrics and pharmacology, and for each subject we had a series of lectures from the consultants. In our third year we would go on to cover eyes, ear nose and throat (ENT), gynaecology and orthopaedics. For me these consultant's lectures were in many ways the highlight of my training. Their lectures were always followed on shortly afterwards by another session on the same topic from one of the tutors, which helped consolidate our learning and sort out anything we were not clear on, as well as emphasizing the nursing aspects. I especially enjoyed medicine, which I found fascinating, and I think this may have been the time when my interest in science really started. That was not a subject I had studied much at school, apart from some biology, as in those days many people still did not really consider it a subject for girls. I was sorry to hear only a few years later that the requirement for consultant's lectures in nurse training was abolished. The idea, I was told at the time was that nursing was a separate profession from medicine and should develop in its own way, but I felt these lectures gave me a better understanding hearing the medical point of view. Also it was to some extent a two way process. We were able to get across to the consultants some of the difficulties or problems we found in caring for their patients.

At the end of our final week of study block we had our second year exams, one paper on each of the four subjects plus an oral exam with the consultant for medicine and surgery. It wasn't long to wait for the results afterwards. I had expected to do reasonably well in medicine and I did, but to my amazement I came out top with high marks in surgery as well. Perhaps I was going to get through my training after all.

Once we had finished our studies for the year it was back on nights. Recently our hours of duty had been reduced again and this had been an opportunity to change the night rotas. Now we worked just 4 nights a week, but covered from 8pm to 8am. This made for a long night, but was worth it to have three nights off. Being in our second year, we knew we were also likely to be given more responsibility and sometimes be the ones who would have to take charge of a ward. I found that rather than being allocated to one ward for the full three months, I was moved a number of times to fill in where needed, and one night I could be the junior and the next one running the ward.

Initially I found myself back on the Children's' Ward working with a staff nurse for a week because another student was off sick. Here, as the junior, I had what was one of the worst jobs I had undertaken so far—the nappies!

There were no disposable nappies then; they were all made of terry towelling. After use they were put to soak in disinfectant in a large bin in the sluice. The junior night nurse then had to take these all out and rinse them in a sink. They had to be completely clean—no stains—before being rung out and put in large bags ready to go to the laundry the next day. If any were not done properly they would be sent back—and you soon heard about it!

After that I was down to the annexe to a non-acute medical ward, to where patients were transferred from the two main medical wards if they needed a longer hospital stay once they were over the acute phase of their illness. It consisted of two wards, one each for men and women, plus a couple of side rooms. A junior night sister was always on duty at the annexe but she spent the nights on another ward, where there was just one student on, and she just came over to the medical ward to check the drugs.

I was on with Jacky Smith, one the nursing auxiliaries. The work was relatively light as almost all the patients were at least to some extent mobile, so we usually got everyone settled for the night in good time. After that we were able to put our feet up and make ourselves comfortable in the day room. Sometimes we were even able to watch a bit of television, kept at low volume, but never for long because transmission closed down before midnight then. A meal was left for us by the day staff, and Jacky heated this up in the ward kitchen at around midnight. We sat together eating in the day room. After that, with little to do, the night could drag. Once we finished reading newspapers and magazines left by patients, we would dose off, but never too deeply. At the sound of a bell or the slightest noise and we would be alerted.

Only a few patients ever needed our attention during the night. There was one man who had a tracheotomy. He was in the side ward nearest to the day room and we were instantly alerted if he started coughing, as that could mean his airway was becoming blocked with mucous. We then had to use the suction apparatus with a fine tube attached to suck his airway clear.

Another was Mrs Strange, a rather nervous woman who had a great difficulty sleeping. She had been moved to a side ward where she would be less disturbed and was written up for a couple of different sleeping tablets, but these seemed to have little effect. She kept ringing her bell and asking for something stronger. Apart from offering her a hot drink there was little I could do. Sister had already been over to check the second dose of tablets and the doctor wouldn't write her up for anything more.

'Just give her some vitamin C,' Sister said when she came round. 'That'll keep her quiet for a while. She can't have any more sleeping pills.'

So, feeling a bit guilty, I gave her a couple of vitamin C tablets. By then I think she had finally got to a state of exhaustion because she took them and promptly fell asleep for the rest of the night. The problem was the next few nights she kept on asking for the 'wonderful pills' that had enabled her to sleep. Unfortunately, and not unsurprisingly, they didn't work the next time she had them.

Another patient was Michael, aged just 22, who suffered from ulcerative colitis. This is a condition where ulcers develop in the large intestine leading to bouts of severe diarrhoea and bleeding. Unfortunately it is a chronic condition and treatment with drugs has limited success. He had already been admitted several times, seriously anaemic and needing a blood transfusion.

'He's being referred to the surgeons,' Sister told me. 'There's nothing more we can do and each time he's readmitted he is worse. He'll need his colon removing.'

'That means he'll have an ileostomy,' I said, aghast. An ileostomy is where the end of the small intestine leads to an opening formed on the abdomen, similar to a colostomy.

'Yes. But he can't go on as he is. At the moment he has no life. He's constantly ill and is in danger of infection or developing an obstruction due to scarring, or even cancer.'

This was true. There's no known cause for this condition and surgery is often the only treatment option left. But the thought of such a young man having an ileostomy for the rest of his life seemed appalling. Unfortunately this is a condition that affects the young.

After the Annexe I could hardly believe it, but I was back on Women's Surgical once again. Here, of course, things were very different and we were lucky to have a chance of sitting down at all. There was one third year there on nights and now I worked opposite her. Working four nights a week meant that we overlapped just one night a week and the next three I was running the ward with a first year. I had mixed feelings starting my first night in charge. On the one hand I looked forward to the challenge and was quite confident I could cope. The night sister, Sister Morrison, was always around to give help and support when needed. But I was not looking forward to having to give the morning report to Sister Lamb after my first night. In the event, in spite of my nervousness, I managed with no criticism from her.

However things did not always go so smoothly. There was one time when I had to fill out the dreaded accident form. This came about because when we had someone due for theatre late in the morning they were sometimes allowed an early cup of tea to be given at 5am. Unfortunately this coincided with the time when one of us would be on our tea break. One night when we had a patient due an early drink, the junior was at her break. I was on my own on the ward, so had to slip out to the kitchen to get the tea. This probably only took a couple of minutes at the most, as everything was ready and, like every ward, we had boiling water on tap from an urn. I had just taken in the tea when I heard a cry from the far end of the ward, from near the toilets. I rushed down to find a patient there, struggling back to her feet. Patients were not supposed to get up at night on their own, but she hadn't wanted to be a bother to us. After all she was up and about during the day, so when she awoke wanting to go to the toilet, she went on her own. Once there she had begun to feel faint and fallen. Luckily she wasn't badly hurt, but had some bruises and a graze on her arm.

I helped her back to bed and gave the graze a clean. Then I had to call night sister and fill in the accident form. This form then went to matron's office and the following night Sister Morrison came to see me.

'Matron wanted to know why you had to leave the ward. I understand that was to get an early tea for another patient.'

'Yes,' I replied. 'We always have to give early teas at 5 am and that's the time when one of us is on our break. We're only out for a moment. It doesn't take long.'

She nodded. 'That's what I thought. It's what I told Matron. I don't know what we can do about it if that is the time it has to be. Also the patient was in the side ward?'

I nodded. The side room was the four bedded ward extending from the bottom of the main ward, very close to the toilets. It was used for patients who were on their way to recovery and able to get up and look after themselves.

'So you mightn't have seen her anyway if you had been attending to someone else.'

That was true. I was glad to feel that I had her support and when I saw her the next night she said that Matron understood and didn't blame me for what had happened.

As usual we also had our share of patients becoming confused during the night. We had one who was determined to get out of bed after having had hip surgery during the day before and, having cot side up, tried to crawl out of the bottom. We could hardly take out eyes off her for a moment without her trying again and we would have to stop what we were doing and restrain her.

There was another lady who could become quite aggressive with us, shouting for attention. On one occasion she demanded a drink of water and, as the junior was giving it to her, she grabbed at the glass so that a small amount spilt around her neck. It wasn't very much, although probably a bit uncomfortable, but she yelled at the nurse, accusing her of pouring water over her. We dried her up and changed her pillowcase, but she continued to accuse us of pouring a glass of water over her and her claim become more and more exaggerated as the night went on. By the morning the glass had become a bucket! She told everyone she could that she had had a bucket of water poured over her. Of course this was obviously untrue and there were plenty of patients as witnesses, but it did worry me a bit. You do hear of older patients in nursing homes complaining of ill treatment. They can simply be confused in an environment strange to them, or perhaps have had a bad dream, but sadly their complaints are sometimes justified. It can therefore be difficult for outsiders to know what's true and what isn't.

Another time after the usual busy night I got back to our house only to meet Kay on the doorstep.

'There's been a call for you from Sister Lamb. She said you've still got the keys.'

My heart sank into my boots. The keys to the medicine cupboard had to be handed over at every change of shift and I had forgotten. They would still be in my uniform pocket in my locker in the Nurses' Home.

'Oh no! How could I have forgotten,' I said. 'All I want to do is go to bed and now I'll have to go all the way back'

Kay grinned, though not unsympathetic. 'You're not the first. I did it on Gynae not so long ago. I forgot to give them to Sister when I went off for the evening and she didn't even notice until the six o'clock drugs were due. It was lucky I hadn't gone out, as I was planning to later.'

Much as I wanted to sleep there was nothing else for it, so back I went to retrieve the keys and take them up to the ward. Sister Lamb was very good about it, almost apologetic, as so she should. After all it had been her fault as much as mine.

13.

Secondment

There was now a big change in store. All of us in my set were seconded for three months to another hospital, one specializing in chest diseases. We were the first set to be seconded there and had been told about it well in advance because we would now all have to live in again. I had to give up my flat sharing with Kay, which I was sorry about, but she would soon be taking her finals and wasn't planning to stay on after that, so I probably wouldn't have stayed there much longer anyway. The hospital where we were going had originally been a sanatorium for TB patients and because of this it was situated well out in the countryside. It did still cater for people with TB, but there were far fewer cases by then, and numbers were still going down, thanks to the availability of the BCG immunization given routinely to all teenagers. Now the hospital catered mainly for people with other kinds of chest conditions, including those needing thoracic surgery.

I started there on one of the medical wards, which included a wing for women with TB. The ward had been built in the days when fresh air was a major part of the treatment. We had just four patients, all in separate rooms with doors facing out onto a covered walkway that was open on the other side. Their views were spectacular, across a valley to open countryside, but bitterly cold during the winter, which was now approaching. In an attempt to provide some shelter the corridor was soon temporarily closed in by tarpaulin sheets with plastic windows for light, which did provide some protection from the worst of the elements, but it was still extremely cold. A couple of times a week the poor patients had their bath day. The bathroom was just as cold as the rest of the ward, with no heating. At least they had hot water for the baths, but afterwards they needed to dry and get dressed as fast as possible.

These patients could expect to be there for several weeks, if not months. They couldn't be discharged until it was certain they were no longer infectious. They had sputum samples collected regularly to check for the presence of the TB organism and this had to be clear before they could go. In the meantime they were being treated with antibiotics specific for the infection, always being given two different drugs at the same time. This was because we were very aware of the danger of the development of drug resistance. If just one type of antibiotic is given there is a risk of the organism becoming resistant to it, but if a second kind of antibiotic is given at the same time, the chances of an organism becoming resistant to both is low, and the treatment will still be effective. Even so today multidrug resistant strains have developed in many countries.

The other half of the ward was, thankfully, indoors. Here there were patients with other chest conditions, such as severe chronic bronchitis or pneumonia. There was also one with empyema, which is an infection within the pleural cavity, the space between the lungs and chest wall, and another young man who had developed a pneumothorax, which is when air escapes into the pleural cavity causing the lung to collapse. These patients had chest drains and I learnt how to prepare and change the drainage bottles. It is important not to let any air to be sucked back up the tube into the pleural cavity, so the tubing had to be clamped off while disconnecting the bottle and attaching a fresh one.

Physiotherapy was a very important part of treating many of these patients. During the weekdays a physiotherapist would visit at least twice a day, using postural drainage by raising the foot of the bed, pummelling the chest wall and getting them to cough. We all had to learn how to do this, since at weekends and nights it was done by nurses. I enjoyed doing it and found it very satisfying when a patient's chest sounded so much clearer afterwards.

As well as the four of us there were two other students seconded there, Carol and Sally, both from Exeter. Together we had more than doubled the number of residents in the Nurses' Home. The only other occupants were the assistant matron, a ward sister and a couple of staff nurses and an enrolled nurse, though we rarely saw any of them—they seemed to keep to their own rooms. We took over the sitting room, which had a record player for our use and that was where we spent most of our evenings off duty. Going out anywhere in the evening was difficult without your own transport as buses to town were slow and infrequent. We were still not allowed a key to the front door, which was locked at 10.30pm. However the trained staff did, and we soon found one of the staff nurses was willing to lend us hers whenever we liked. Furthermore there were no strict rules about visitors. Carol had a boyfriend who seemed to spend most evenings there with us in the sitting room. Whether he got any further than that I never knew.

One night I had been out with Sally to a party in Exeter and by the time we got back it was around 1am. We had been dropped off by her boyfriend at the Nurses' Home and crept in as quietly as we could. Her room was on the first floor and I whispered goodnight to her as I went on up to the floor above, as my room was on the second (top) floor. It was the first room you came to at the top of the stairs on the landing. Just beyond it the corridor narrowed. As I approached my room to my horror I heard a door further down the corridor open and someone come out. I knew this was the assistant matron.

I froze, not sure what to do. I was hidden from her view, but if I rummaged in my bag for my room key and unlocked the door she was certain to hear. But if she walked down the corridor she would see me. I took the risk and stood silently by my door, praying that she wouldn't come along the corridor and see me hiding. Thankfully she didn't, but just crossed the corridor to the toilets. As soon as she was in there I unlocked my door and got into my room as fast as possible. I don't know what she would have said if she had found me. Perhaps not a lot, but she would have wanted to know where I got the key from. The staff nurse who had lent it to us would have been in trouble and we wouldn't have been able to borrow it again.

One evening towards the end of our stay some of us were together in the sitting room when Carol said 'I want to get my ears pierced.'

'I've thought about that too,' said Pat. 'You can wear far nicer earrings for pierced ears, and clip on ones pinch.'

It was something I had thought about too, but when it came to it I was too much of a coward to have it done.

But Carol went on. 'It must be really easy to do. All you need is a bit of local anaesthetic and a needle. Why waste money when you can do it yourself. I'm going to do it, but I may want one of you to help.'

None of us expected her to go through with it, but the next evening she came down to the sitting room with some of the local anaesthetic spray that we used on patients, some surgical spirit and needles, all borrowed from the ward, and some new sleepers ready to put in afterwards.

'Well, who's going to help me?' she asked.

'You're not really going to do it?' Hilary voiced what we were all thinking.

'Of course I am. But it will be much easier if someone helps.'

I was having nothing to do with it, but she was determined, and eventually Sally gave way. 'There's no way you can do it on your own. If you're certain about it then I'll do it for you. But say if you want me to stop.'

'Good. We need to sterilize the sleepers first. I've got a galipot for that.' She produced a small metal bowl, again borrowed from the ward. She put in the sleepers and covered them with spirit.

'I've marked where I think they should go.' She showed us where she had made a small pen mark on each ear lobe.

'OK, let me spray them,' said Sally. She sprayed each ear with a good amount of local anaesthetic. We waited for it to have an effect.

'I can still feel them.' Carol said, pinching her ear lobes with her fingers.

'I'll use a bit more spray.'

Now they seemed to be numb and after cleaning them with spirit, Sally used a large needle and pierced the first ear. Carol flinched slightly.

'Did you feel it?'

'A bit. But carry on.'

Sally managed to insert the sleeper. One ear was done.

'I think I need a bit more local for the other one.' It had obviously been painful so Sally used more spray.

'Are you sure you want me to go on?'

'Well you can't stop now. I can't have just one pierced ear.'

Sally completed the second ear and Carol inspected the result in the mirror which hung over the fireplace.

'It looks really good,' she exclaimed. She looked more closely. 'Are the even? I think this one is a bit lower than the other.'

We all looked. They were definitely not quite level. 'There's hardly any difference,' I reassured her. 'It won't be noticeable, especially when you have proper earrings in.'

She seemed happy with that.

So the operation was a success and two or three weeks later Carol appeared wearing a pair of long dangly earrings.

After the first four weeks I was moved to the surgical ward for the remaining two months of my secondment. Here all the rooms lead off a main corridor, which was reported to be a quarter of a mile long, making it the longest ward any of us had ever known. Since it took about five minutes walking fast to get from one end to the other I think this estimate was probably correct.

Many of the patients here were in for investigation following X-rays that had revealed tumours in the lungs; suspected lung cancer. They were mostly men, since women didn't smoke so much in those days, although their numbers were increasing. But there was one woman I remember who was still only in her thirties. She had smoked heavily from her teens and now it was confirmed that she had developed lung cancer. It was too far advanced to be treated and she did not take the news well. She wanted to blame someone so she blamed it on the medical profession, who she said should have stopped her from smoking.

It was only the previous decade that Professor Doll had made the link between smoking and cancer. This had received a tremendous amount of publicity, so she must have known, although she would have already been a smoker by then. I don't know if anyone, such as her GP, had ever advised her to stop, but I suspect she would have been resistant to the advice if they had. Of course we realised that she was looking for someone else to blame because she was angry, as well she might. After all it did seem so unfair when many smokers go on to a ripe old age.

It was surprising that the link to cancer had so little effect on the numbers of smokers. Of course it is an addiction so it can be extremely hard to stop, but the numbers taking it up also continued to rise. I found that, when presented with the evidence, smokers seemed to divide into two main groups; the deniers and the fatalists. The deniers refused to believe the evidence and the fatalists said 'well, you have to die of something'.

None of our set smoked, although quite a lot of nurses did. I had certainly tried, but the main thing that put me off was the expense. I worked out how much it would cost to smoke just ten a day for a week, then a month and then a year. I decided straight away that I could find something much better to spend my hard earned money on. Even if I had taken it up I think I would have been put off after nursing patients who were smokers. Although lung cancer was now receiving all the attention, just as bad are the many other lung conditions like chronic bronchitis, which can lead to heart failure, also linked to smoking. Also after surgery I found the smokers frequently developed nasty chesty coughs as a result of the anaesthetic. They had to be encouraged to cough to keep their chest clear, but it is extremely painful to cough when you have stitches.

To make a diagnosis patients with suspected lung cancer would have to undergo a bronchoscopy, whereby a long metal tube is passed down the throat and into the lungs so that a biopsy of the tumour can be taken. I was sent with one of the patients, a man in his fifties, to watch. No general anaesthetic was given, so the patient was awake throughout, but his throat numbed. The front of his neck was sprayed with local anaesthetic, and then local anaesthetic injected into his throat from there. For the tube to be passed the patient had to lie on his back with his head extended backwards. In spite of the local anaesthetic I thought the whole procedure looked extremely unpleasant. Afterwards the patient was not allowed to eat or drink until the local anaesthetic had worn off in case he choked.

The surgery carried out to remove a tumour might involve removal of part or even the whole of one lung, and this operation might also be done for other lung diseases, not just cancer. After surgery they would be nursed in the room next to the office and would need what we called 'specialing', which is when one nurse stays with them all the time for the first few hours. They would come back to the ward with a multitude of tubes and drains attached, including at least one intravenous infusion, usually blood, chest drains, a catheter, and would still have an airway in place until they regained consciousness. They might need observations taken as frequently as every five minutes at first, so you would be kept busy.

The ward sister there was lovely. She always had time to show us how things were done, such as shortening and removing chest drains. However none of us got on with one of the staff nurses who I had already heard much about before starting on the surgical wards. I don't know what her problem was—perhaps she disliked students for some reason, but she was extremely unpleasant and just plain rude in the way she ordered us around. The others seemed to put up with it, although all felt resentment at their treatment, but I am never very tolerant of this sort of behaviour.

I couldn't believe she was as bad as the others had said and was on the ward for a week or so before I first had to work with her as she had been on holiday. She soon lived up to her reputation and over the next few days I felt increasingly angry at her attitude. One evening we had a patient arriving back from theatre and I was to look after him. Two doctors, including the anaesthetist, came to the ward with him and, after we transferred him to his bed, we began organizing all the various tubes. Staff nurse was behaving in her usual way, ordering me to do something else before I had finished what she had already told me to do. I was still doing his observations, taking his blood pressure when she was ordering me to do something else.

I felt as though I was going to snap, so as calmly as I could I said 'I can only do one thing at a time, so I will do it when I have finished this.'

She was silent for a moment, unable to believe someone had answered her back.

Finally she spoke to the anaesthetist. 'Did you hear what she said?'

He didn't say anything, but I am sure the corners of his mouth were twitching.

She said nothing more and finally left me alone to get on with caring for the patient. I was thinking, oh dear, I'm probably going to get into trouble now. She is sure to complain and will be even worse than ever with me now. Perhaps I should apologize. But no, I had been fully justified in saying what I did and hadn't exactly been rude. Rather surprisingly nothing more was said. In fact after that she was always extremely polite and seemed almost nervous of me. She clearly couldn't cope with anyone who stood up to her in any way.

By the end of our three months we had all learnt a lot, especially as our ward work had been complemented by a course of weekly study days. I think we all enjoyed our time there, but were pleased when it was time for us to return to our own hospital.

14.

Third year

'I've passed, I've passed!' I greeted Hilary as I returned from days off. No, it wasn't a nursing exam, but my driving test. I had nearly cancelled the test because I had missed lessons due to snow and thought I needed more practice, but then thought I might as well take it as a trial run. Probably because of this I was more relaxed and somehow managed to pass. I think even my driving instructor was a bit surprised. The following week, with my father's help and advice, I bought a rather old Morris Minor at the cost of £100. I had to buy it on what was then known as HP, or hire purchase, with £20 down and paying off the £80 loan over the next year. Getting a loan like this was frowned upon by some people in those days, but it was the only way I could afford it and I was determined to pay it off as quickly as possible. Now I was much more independent and didn't have to rely on buses crawling through the Devon lanes when I visited home, which involved two changes, and it would certainly advance my social life.

Hilary and I were now sharing a flat. It was very close to the hospital, so much so that we often walked to work, even though we both had cars. This was quite unusual as not many student nurses had cars then. Luckily our landlady, who lived on the ground floor below our flat, didn't have a car herself, and there was just room for them both in the driveway. Whenever I did drive to work, there was no difficulty parking there either; there was usually space in the court yard directly in front of the hospital main building.

Mrs Dowson, our landlady, was a well built woman in her late sixties and quite a character. We all got on well and she would sometimes invite us in to tea with her, but never imposed herself on us. Shortly after we got the flat Pat and Nancy came over after work one evening and stayed quite late. We downed a bottle of wine and listened to the latest Beatles album on my new record player. If Hilary had been there I am sure she would have told us to keep the noise down a bit and the next day I was worried that we might have disturbed Mrs Dowson. I saw her as I got back the following evening, so thought I should say something.

'I hope we didn't disturb you too much last night,' I said. 'I know we were up rather late.'

'Last night? No I didn't hear anything. I wasn't wearing my hearing aid.'

She had been married three times, she told us, and her ex's had been disposed of in various ways, one died and the others divorced – and she hadn't given up on the idea of there being a husband number four. Two or three times a year she would take herself off on coach tours to different parts of the country. After one of these she told us that a gentleman she had met would be coming to stay. Perhaps this would be number four. He duly arrived and seemed pleasant enough when we met him rather briefly. After he left we were invited in to tea and we went looking forward to hearing more. It turned out he had been a disappointment.

'He was really quite selfish,' she told us. 'Every day I always asked him how his hip was doing, but he never once asked me about my arthritis.'

So he wasn't seen again. A couple or so years later, after we had both left, I found out that she had actually remarried and gone to live in Totnes. She did not outlive this husband.

Now in our third year we sported smart new maroon belts, replacing our grey ones. I remembered when we had first started, how the third year students seemed so impossibly experienced and knowledgeable. There were only a few specialities left where I still hadn't worked, but I started off on the Private Ward, which I never really enjoyed. Sister Phelps was in charge, always immaculately groomed with blond hair and a hint of subtly applied make up. She spent most of her time in the office talking to consultants, just coming out to do rounds of the patients. I did not find her very approachable.

Most patients came in with relatively minor complaints, perhaps for routine surgery, and much of the time there was relatively little to do. When I first started I was told by Sister Phelps that here we had 'time to concentrate on the finer points of nursing', which might be true, but I felt rather guilty that I had so little to do when I knew how rushed everyone was on other wards, where we could barely get through the essential work. Here, instead of the time flying by, the days dragged. Some mornings I would perhaps have one patient to bed bath and a couple of dressings and could finish these tasks by mid morning, after which I still had an hour or so to go until lunch. On some days we might have a patient for theatre who needed preparing and would have to be checked regularly for a while afterwards. Otherwise patients were all behind closed doors and didn't want to be disturbed. I spent a considerable amount of time 'tidying the sluice' and trying to find anything that needed restocking in the treatment room. The afternoons were worse since they would all have visitors, although at least the visitors brought in plenty of flowers, so I was able to take my time in arranging them. When Sister was off and one of the Staff Nurses left in charge it was much more relaxed and we were able to sit in the office, just getting up if someone rang a bell.

I remember one patient, a girl of about my age, who had come in to have a mole removed from her back, mainly for cosmetic reasons. She was clearly very nervous and fussed over everything as I prepared her for theatre. I had to control my impatience, and tried to tell myself that I would have been just as nervous if it had been me, even if it was a minor procedure. But it made me realise how much I preferred being in the thick of it, dealing with emergencies and caring for the seriously ill.

In spite of my boredom though, all the patients were extremely pleasant, and I enjoyed my conversations with them when I had the chance. I had thought that, as they were paying for their treatment, they would be much more demanding and aloof. I commented on this to Staff Nurse.

'Oh yes,' she said. 'We have had several 'Lady' or 'Sir' this and that, since I've been here and they have all been lovely people. The more upper class they are the nicer they seem to be. We do get some difficult customers though, but interestingly they tend to be the ones who have just come into money, or perhaps have got medical insurance through their job. They are the ones who seem to think they should be waited on hand and foot.'

'Still I suppose you get people like that anywhere,' I said, thinking of one or two difficult customers I had come across on the wards.

Attached to the private wing was the nurses' sick bay, a two bedded room, which had been empty most of my time there—until my final week when Kathy was brought in.

Kathy had developed a severe headache over a couple of days. She couldn't eat and had been vomiting. All she wanted to do was lie there and sleep with the curtains drawn. Her temperature was only very slightly raised and otherwise her observations were normal. I was there when the consultant came to examine her. It was usual for consultants to see staff who were admitted rather than the more junior housemen.

'Have you any pain?' he asked.

She gave a brief nod.

'Where is the pain?'

With an effort she tried to move her arm, but only got her hand as far as her chest.

He continued with his examination, testing her for neck stiffness—there was perhaps a little, looking into her eyes, listening to her chest and examining her abdomen. There wasn't anything obviously abnormal.

Afterwards Sister told me to collect a urine sample from her for the laboratory.

'She may just have a urinary tract infection,' she told me.

I didn't think that very likely, but of course it would have to be ruled out. With some difficulty I got her up and to the toilet, and managed to get a sample from her. It was all I could do to keep her awake long enough to provide it in the requisite container.

'She must eat something,' Sister said to me after that. 'You take her supper in and make sure she eats it.'

I went in with her tray, but although I sat her up with her plate in front and handed her a knife and fork, it was clear she couldn't feed herself. I tried to feed her, but she wouldn't swallow. As I talked to her I realised that she didn't even seem to know who I was. I went back to Sister.

'She won't eat anything.' I hesitated, and then went on. 'She's getting worse. There's her headache and she can't stand daylight—she's photophobic—and she's becoming confused. Those are cerebral symptoms.'

For a moment I thought she was going to be annoyed with me as she paused before speaking.

'I agree. I will talk to the doctor again.'

That night Kathy was transferred to the regional neurological centre in Bristol where she was diagnosed with encephalitis, an infection of the brain. There, with the proper treatment, she made a slow recovery and, after a few weeks, was able to go home to Scotland for a prolonged convalescence. I hoped we would all see her back again soon, but it wasn't going to be for a few months.

Kathy wasn't the only one who was unwell. Hilary hadn't been feeling too good for a while. She had had several episodes when her temperature had been up a bit, only to settle again. Then one day her temperature was much higher and she felt awful. She went to see Home Sister, who put her in the sick bay next to her office in the nurses' home. That evening Miss Vernon, the assistant matron, visited her when doing her rounds and Hilary told her how her temperature had been high the previous evening.

'What are you doing taking you own temperature?' Miss Vernon demanded. 'It is not your business. You should come to home sister if you don't feel well and she will do whatever is necessary.'

Hilary could hardly believe it, but this exemplified the attitude of some, mostly older, staff at this time. Patients were not always given full information about their condition, although it might be discussed with near relatives. They were expected to do as they were told and not ask questions; in other word 'doctor knows best'. Many of us didn't go along with this attitude and if anyone wanted to know what their temperature was I would certainly tell them, but not everyone would.

Hilary was eventually diagnose with glandular fever and was off sick for a few weeks. When she returned to work she was worried.

'I can't be off sick again for more than two days,' she told me. 'If I'm off more than that I won't have done enough training to take my finals next February and I'll have to wait another four months and take it with the next set.'

By then we had about six months training to go, so we all hoped she would make it.

15.

Specialities and Maternity

I was glad to move on, to ENT (ear, nose and throat) and them, rather briefly, to the eye ward. ENT was a calm and well ordered ward. Most of the patients were in for relatively minor routine surgery, such as sinus washouts and children having their tonsils removed, quite a common operation then. Children who had this operation were given soluble aspirin gargles before meals and then fed ice cream to sooth their sore throats. Most of the work was routine and I was only sorry that I never got to syringe any ears during my short time there.

The only really sick patient while I was there was Mr Gordon, who had developed cancer of his larynx (voice box) and came in to have this removed. After the operation he would have a permanent tracheotomy and not be able to speak normally. It seemed a really drastic operation, but Sister assured me that he would be able to learn to speak again.

'We have got Jack coming in to see him this afternoon,' she told me. 'You must go and have a word with him.'

Jack, it turned out, had had this operation a few years before and had learnt to speak by swallowing air and then managed to form a few word as the air was regurgitated. I could hardly imagine how anyone could do this, but when Jack came in he spoke perfectly clearly, if rather hesitantly, as he could only manage a few words before having to pause to gulp down more air. His visit certainly did a lot to reassure Mr Gordon, who went on to have the operation successfully. He still couldn't speak by the time he went home as that was going to take a bit of time, but he was determined to succeed so I hope it all went well for him.

In the eye ward patients were all in rooms of between two to four beds, with men and women in separate rooms of course—no mixed sex wards then. One of the most common eye operations was removing cataracts. There were no artificial lenses available then to insert in its place, so afterwards patients needed strong glasses. They were kept in hospital for at least three or four days after their operation. Immediately afterwards they would always have someone sitting with them for the first few hours, making certain they didn't rub the affected eye while they were still drowsy from their anaesthetic. After that they were nursed lying flat for up to 48 hours and we had to do everything for them, even feed them. Their eye drops were always left for Sister to do the first time and she liked to do most of them when she was on duty, but at other times it was often my job. Contrast this with today where cataracts are done as outpatients, with patients going home around 4 hours later.

The maternity ward was somewhere I had been hoping to get the chance to work, so was please when I was allocated there. This would give me an idea as to whether or not I should go on to do midwifery training after qualifying. It was a small consultant unit where mothers were delivered if they had, or were thought to be at risk of developing, any complications of normal pregnancy and childbirth. At this time most babies were born at home or in small maternity units in some of the surrounding towns where they would be under the care of their GP. Any mothers who developed complications were transferred here.

Women tended to be kept in bed far longer than now after childbirth. Not so long before it could be up to a week, but we had become aware of the possible dangers of this practice, mainly that of deep vein thrombosis (DVT) due to inactivity, and now we got them up after 24 hours, still much later than today. The babies were kept separately in the nursery and would just be taken out to their mothers for feeding. I enjoyed having to change their nappies before taking them to their mothers and giving out bottles to anyone not breast feeding. Those needing help with breast feeding were attended to by one of the midwives.

Many mothers and babies were transferred to GP units a couple of days after giving birth if this was nearer to their home, otherwise they could stay in hospital for about eight days. Before they went home we had to make sure the babies were feeding well and gaining weight, and the mothers knew how to change their nappies and bath them. All nappies were made of terry towelling, and first time mothers needed quite a bit of practice learning how to fold these and get them to fit the tiny babies without them falling off. One of my favourite jobs was carrying the baby down to the car when a husband came to take his wife and newborn home, although many mothers and babies were taken home by ambulance as not so many people owned cars then.

Side wards were used for anyone in labour or for the first day or so after having a caesarean section. There was just one delivery room, and if they were busy with more than one mother in labour, they had to use a side room for deliveries as well.

I was longing to see a birth. They were never shown on TV in those days, so I didn't really know what to expect, but I had to wait for a few days because they all seemed to happen during the night. Then one day when I came on duty I was told that a Mrs Luscombe had been admitted in labour. She was progressing well and I should go and help the staff midwife, Pam Milner, who was looking after her. Husbands didn't stay to be present at deliveries then and Mr Luscombe had been sent home with instructions to phone later, so I joined Pam to sit with his wife. Mrs Luscombe seemed in an awful lot of pain, and I was shown how to help her with using the gas and air machine. It seemed to take a dreadfully long time, but eventually she began to get the urge to push, indicating that her cervix was fully dilated and she was in the second stage. We moved her into the labour ward.

It was her first baby and I was told that the second stage could last for up to two hours. Now we urged her to push with her contractions and the midwife checked the foetal heart regularly using a small trumpet shaped instrument; the foetal stethoscope—no monitors then.

'That's fine,' she said. 'A good strong heart beat. Look, you can just see the top of baby's head.'

I looked, and there it was, just visible, but still with a way to go. Unfortunately, in spite of the mother's valiant efforts, that was where it stayed. After over an hour of pushing it was clear that no progress was being made and Mrs Luscombe was exhausted.

'I'm afraid it's stuck there,' said Pam. 'I'll have to let the doctor know. Don't worry,' she spoke to the mother, 'It looks like you need a bit of help. We'll soon have baby out.'

The doctor arrived and we prepared for a forceps delivery. I was shown how to lift her legs up to go in stirrups so that the doctor could deliver the baby. He washed her down with antiseptic and draped her with sterile towels. The he injected local anaesthetic using a very long needle to numb the birth canal. Once this had taken effect he got out the forceps. I watched in horror as these were inserted, one blade at a time, in and around the baby's head. I couldn't believe that anything that big could actually fit in there!

With next contraction Mrs Luscombe was encouraged to push as the doctor pulled, and in no time the head was delivered, shortly followed by the rest of the baby.

'It's a boy.'

The baby was crying lustily and the midwife showed him to his delighted and relieved mother. He was then put in a cot while the doctor finished off, delivering the placenta and then stitching up the episiotomy, the cut he had made to help the delivery of the baby's head.

'Don't the forceps hurt the baby?' I asked the midwife afterwards. 'The doctor had to pull really hard.'

She laughed. 'No, a lot of people think that, but they shouldn't put any pressure of the baby's head. They actually protect it. We often use forceps for premature births, where the bones of the skull are much softer, just for that reason. Look,'

She showed me the forceps that had been used, now washed off.

'When the handles are together the blades can't meet. They fit around the head. When the doctor pulls, he is pulling against the birth canal, opening it to allow the baby's head through.'

I could see what she meant and had a go fitting the blades together.

Next she showed me the placenta, which she had already examined carefully to make sure it was complete.

'It usually comes out all in one piece,' she told me, 'but occasionally a bit can be left behind. Even a small bit can be enough to cause a serious bleed later—that's a post partum haemorrhage—so it's important to check carefully.'

After Mrs Luscombe had enjoyed the traditional cup of tea, I gave her a wash before moving her back to bed in the ward. Pam now bathed the baby.

'We always leave them to rest for an hour before giving them their bath,' she explained. 'They have been through a lot, so need to recover before we start disturbing them again.'

The forceps delivery had been a bit of a shock to me, but the next delivery I witnessed was a normal one, and I saw several more during my time there. I often thought the whole business of labour and delivery was enough to put anyone off the thought of childbirth for the rest of their life, but there is nothing quite like the feeling you get when at last you are holding the new born baby. Sometimes I was able to give the baby its first bath and I always enjoyed getting them cleaned up, washing and brushing their hair—if they had any—and dressing them for the first time. They always wore hospital clothes, just vests and jackets with their nappies. Their own clothes were brought in later and they were changed into these to go home.

Some of the mothers seemed very young. One was having her second child at just eighteen, younger than me. Even so all mothers were addressed as 'Mrs so and so', never Christian names then. I only remember one unmarried mother and she gave up her baby for adoption, much more commonly done then. Her baby son was taken away immediately after birth and she didn't handle him at all. He remained in the nursery and we looked after him until he was collected by a social worker to go to his adoptive parents. His mother was kept in a side ward after the birth so that she wouldn't see all the other mothers with their babies, but she would certainly have heard them. She never said anything much, always very quiet and I didn't really know what to say to her. She must have found it all terrible.

I was glad of the experience I got on the maternity ward, especially since I now felt that I would have some idea how to deliver a baby in an emergency; something all nurses should be able to do. I thought I would enjoy delivering babies, so perhaps I would do midwifery training later, but probably should get a bit of experience as a staff nurse first.

16.

Final year nights

The weather was glorious, Casualty was busy treating holiday makers with sunburn, and we were back on nights. The morning after the first night I met Nancy in the changing room after coming off duty.

'It's too nice out to spend the day in bed,' she said. 'It'll probably be too hot to sleep anyway—I feel hot already. I'd love to go for a swim.'

'Why don't we,' I suggested. 'If we bring our swimming things in with us tonight, tomorrow morning we could. I've got the car, so we can go to one of the beaches away from the crowds. Not that it'll be crowded first thing.'

So that's what we did, not just the next day, but several times over the next month when we were both on the same nights. We went to the beach in Babbacombe at the foot of the funicular railway, had a swim, and lazed in the sun to dry off until around midday. I was a bit worried that we would fall asleep and lie there for too long in the sun, but we never did. Once we got back to our respective flats we both slept better the rest of the day for it.

I was now on Men's Surgical, probably the busiest ward in the hospital and somewhere I had been looking forward to working, although was a bit apprehensive as to how I would cope. The first few nights I was on with Staff Nurse Merrifield, who worked permanently on nights and later I covered her nights off. Like the Women's Surgical, it took both surgical and accident cases and it wasn't uncommon to have two or three emergency admissions in a night. They could be for things like acute appendicitis or bowel obstructions, which I had been used to dealing with on

Women's Surgical, as well as victims of road accidents. These were mainly young motorcyclists, and their most common injury was a fractured femur, although head and back injuries were also common. I began to really dislike motor cycles. For a fractured femur they would go to theatre to have a metal pin inserted through the lower end of the bone just above their knee, and traction would be applied to this. Staff Nurse Merrifield showed me how to set this up. It was important, she told me, to shave the leg first, before applying the sticking plaster; otherwise it would be very painful when it came to its removal later. These young men were all put together at the far end of the ward and, once they had recovered from the initial trauma, they could be somewhat lively!

Head injuries were also common and we had to monitor them very carefully in case there was any bleeding beneath the skull. If this happened they would need urgent treatment to relieve the pressure on the brain. We didn't do neurosurgery there, which was all the more reason to be vigilant as, if they did need surgery, they would have to be transferred all the way to Bristol. We had one young man who had seemed to be recovering well the first night after he was admitted, but had become steadily more disorientated and drowsy during the following evening. When I came on duty I was shocked to see the change in him and was relieved when he was transferred to Bristol, where he was operated on successfully.

Another young man who was with us for a number of weeks was Simon. Once again his injuries were due to a motor cycle accident, and it was not the first time. He had been in the year before with a fractured femur. Now he'd damaged his spine. To prevent injury to his spinal cord, which could have led to paralysis, he had to be kept absolutely flat. Of course he still needed turning to prevent pressure sores, so he was nursed in a special spinal bed. When he was on his back, to turn him over, another piece of the bed was put over him and this was strapped firmly round the bottom, so that he was sandwiched between the two parts. This was then turned over so that what had been at the bottom was at the top and could be removed. He was now lying prone. There was a hole for his face, looking down towards the floor, so that he didn't have to turn his head. He had to be turned over in this way every two hours, so two hours later he was turned back. The bottom piece had a section that could be removed if he needed a bedpan.

Patients weren't allowed to smoke in the ward of course, not just because we had oxygen cylinders in use, but because of the dangers of smoking in bed. Nevertheless we did sometimes find sheets and blankets with scorch marks and even holes burnt through them. On this ward smoking was restricted to the day room which as a result always reeked of tobacco smoke. After surgery many men made it there as soon as possible afterwards to get their fix, but the motor cycle boys, as the motor cycle accident victims were often known, were more restricted when they were on traction. If we had time we sometimes wheeled them in their beds out to the day room, and back when they had finished their smoke, before settling them for the night. Lack of anywhere to smoke didn't seem to be such a problem on women's wards, largely because far fewer women smoked then.

Apart from accidents a frequent cause for admission was acute retention of urine as a result of an enlarged prostate gland, a common problem for older men. These men would be in extreme pain from their distended bladder and would have to have a catheter inserted to relieve the obstruction. Later they would need surgery to remove their prostate gland and prevent a recurrence. After this operation they would have to have their bladder washed out regularly via their catheter to prevent it getting blocked with blood, and keeping it clear could take a good deal of our time. Doctors always did male catheterizations then, while nurses did female. This wasn't just that female catheterization is easier, which it isn't always, but then virtually all doctors were men and nurses women, so it was rather less embarrassing for the patients. Things are different now, and many nurses do learn how to catheterize men.

A further problem that can occur within the urinary system is the formation of kidney stones. When they move they can block the ureters, which normally drain urine from the kidney to the bladder. Urine backs up in the kidneys causing the extreme pain known as renal colic. This has been described as the worst pain known to man—but not to woman as for them it's childbirth. The stones may eventually pass through the system, but if they don't and they cause more trouble, they may need removing surgically. We had one man in his twenties who was admitted for surgery the next day after having had a couple of severe bouts of renal colic. The ward was particularly busy when I came on duty. We had a couple of emergency admissions, another patient who was confused and noisy, plus the motor cycle boys were in a boisterous mood. The poor man must have thought it was a madhouse. I had finally got things more settled and turned the lights down for the night when I found him up and dressed. He had decided he had had enough and was off home. I called Night Sister and we tried to persuade him to stay, but he had made up his mind and signed the discharge form. I felt sorry that he had seen the ward at its worst. For someone unused to hospitals it must have been unsettling. Whether he ever had his kidney stones removed I never found out.

There were inevitably some tragic cases. One was a young man who had been brought in during the evening seriously injured after a road accident, but had died on the ward shortly before we came on for the night. His parents were in London and had left home to travel down here after being told of the accident. Staff Nurse had managed to contact them at Paddington Station by getting a call put out for them over the loud speakers. After receiving the news of his death they decided to travel down anyway. I was glad that I didn't have to deal with all this. Night Sister would see them when they arrived and take them to the mortuary to see their son if they wished.

Another time we had a man in his thirties who had attempted to commit suicide by shooting himself with a rifle. It's not too easy to do this and, although he had tried to aim it at his heart, he had missed and the bullet went through his abdomen instead. He had been suffering from depression for some time and he told Sister that, when he realised he had missed, he wanted to try again, but couldn't bring himself to do it as the first shot had been so painful. The bullet had damaged part of his bowel and he underwent an operation where part of his colon and small intestine were removed and the remainder stitched back together again. The trouble with such an injury to the gut is that its content isn't sterile and this contaminates the peritoneum, the abdominal cavity that contains all the gut. In spite of him being given antibiotics, peritonitis set in and after a couple of weeks he died. I suppose that was what he wanted, but it was such an unpleasant way to die.

In spite of all this we did have some fun during the night. It was rare to go through a night without seeing the doctor on call at some stage, and he usually looked in last thing to check if there was anything that needed doing before trying to settle for the night. These junior doctors, the housemen, could sometimes be up all or most of the night if there were several emergencies, and they still had to work the next day doing the routine ward rounds and clinics. Often they hadn't had time to stop for meals during the day, so we would make them omelettes and toast and mugs of coffee in the ward kitchen. We did try not to call them more than really necessary during the night, but of course we did sometimes have to.

I had really enjoyed my three months there on nights and the challenge of being in charge. I found I got on well with Staff Nurse Merrifield on the nights we worked together. It was a nice change to have some nights working as the junior. Towards the end of my three months I was on with her one night when it was not too busy, and we were sitting and talking quietly.

'Can I tell you something,' she said, 'but don't tell anyone else. I don't want them to know just yet, but I will be leaving sometime early next year.'

'What are you going to do?' I asked.

'Well I've been here almost two years and I really think I've done enough nights. I'm getting a job on days. I'm going back to Southampton, where I trained, and if I get a bit more experience there I will be looking for a sister's post. There doesn't seem to be a chance of that here. Sisters only seem to leave if they retire.'

That was true. There had only been two changes of ward sister within the hospital during my training. I thought for a moment and then said.

'You couldn't do me a favour? When you give in your notice, could you let me know? I've been wondering where I want to work when I finish training and I'd really like to work here. If I can ask as soon as there's a vacancy I might be able to.'

She promised me she would let me know.

17.

The pool

One of the things we always dreaded was when, shortly after coming on duty, you got a call from Matron's office to say someone had gone off sick and another ward was short of staff, so you were to go there to help out. Just as you had got your work organized you had to go and start again somewhere else. Some nurses really resented this and grumbled that we shouldn't have to do it, but most of us saw that there really was little option. However now during our training it had been decided that we should all spend six weeks in what was known as 'The Pool'. There would be around half a dozen of us at any one time, covering both days and nights, and we could be used wherever we were most needed.

This was what I found myself doing next. Our off duty rota for the week was posted on the notice board outside Matron's office and this was where we had to go when coming on duty every day to find out where we were to be for that shift. I don't think any of us enjoyed the pool very much; there was no continuity. If you were very lucky you could spend a few days or nights on the same ward, but often it was somewhere different every shift and you could be moved again to somewhere else at any time.

I seemed to be somewhere different every day. When nowhere was especially short of staff I would be sent to the Private Ward, where we were expected to give the patients extra attention. I remembered my time there earlier in the year when Kathy had been admitted, so ill. Then, on my second day there, who should walk in but Kathy herself.

'You're back!' I exclaimed. 'How are you? It's good to see you again.'

'It's good to be back. I've missed everyone so much.'

'We've missed you too. How long have you been here? Have you just started?'

'Yes. This is my first day back. It all seems very strange. You know I can't remember anything about being ill here. But I am much better now and they're going to see how I get on. They've put me here to work because it's quiet and easier. But I'm not sure what I'm supposed to do. I can't remember how to do anything.'

'Don't worry. I am here for a day or two, so ask just me.'

But she was right when she said she couldn't remember. I had to show her how to do even the simplest things, such as taking temperatures. Luckily there was plenty of time for me to do this but after a couple of days inevitably I was moved on to another ward. Not long afterwards I found out from Tess that Kathy hadn't been able to cope and had had to leave permanently. It was sad because she had been so keen to be able to nurse.

One day when I came on to a late shift Miss Norris, one of the assistant matrons, took me to one side.

'We have a patient who came in last night. You may have heard about her,' she said. I knew immediately who she meant, word had spread rapidly. This woman had attempted suicide by pouring petrol over herself and setting it alight. She was still alive, but had over 80% burns, and it was then considered impossible to recover from anything over about 50%. So it was just a matter of time and trying to make her as comfortable as possible for as long as she remained alive.

'She needs someone to special her. She can't be left, but I can't put a junior nurse in with her and there's no staff nurse available. Are you alright to do it?'

I nodded. 'Yes, of course I'll do it.'

I had never seen anyone with serious burns before, let alone nursed them. Normally such patients would be sent to a specialized unit elsewhere, but as she was beyond treatment it had been decided not to subject her to a lengthy journey and to keep her here.

It was with some apprehension that I made my way to the ward where she was being nursed, in a single room that was normally part of the eye ward. The first thing I noticed when I entered the room was the smell; a mixture of burnt flesh and hair, and petrol. She was a large lady, still in her thirties. Her flesh was blackened and raw where the full thickness of the skin was destroyed. The only parts of her unaffected were her feet and ankles, since the flames had gone upwards, and she was just covered with a sheet, being unable to wear a nightgown.

The main effect of severe burns is shock as a result of loosing fluid from the exposed area where there is no intact skin covering. The fluid loss would be plasma, not just blood, which would mean she was losing protein and electrolytes and this would affect the function of every organ of the body. Already her lungs were filling with fluid and, because she couldn't wear an oxygen mask, she was in an oxygen tent to help her breathing. She was having morphine for pain, which must have been excruciating, although where burns are full skin thickness the nerve ending are destroyed, so these areas would be numb. Later there would be a high risk of infection setting in, but no one expected her to survive long enough for that.

There was little I could do but to sit there. It was difficult to do any observations, but they weren't really necessary. I took her pulse, which I did by feeling her jugular vein in her neck as her wrists were so raw, but that was all. But later she became very restless and panicking, unable to get her breath. She was becoming confused and started to try to pull down the oxygen tent, not realising it was there to help her. I had to get hold of her wrists to restrain her and I remember some of the flesh coming off in my hands. Later she became quieter and weaker. I was glad when my shift ended and I could hand over to someone else.

I never really found out why she did what she did; only that she had had a row with someone, a man friend I think. No one came to visit her while I was there, but perhaps anyone wanting to see her had been dissuaded considering her condition. I can't imagine a much worse way to attempt suicide. Today it is possible that she could have survived as, due to improved treatments, some people have been known to survive with up to 90% burns, but had she survived she would have been dreadfully scarred. As it was she died a day later.

While in the pool we all had to do a couple of weeks on nights and I began my turn with a week on Children's Ward where the staff nurse was on holiday, so I was the senior nurse on duty. I was probably more nervous about this than I had ever been on any of the adult wards, knowing how precious each one of my charges was to their families. Giving children their medicines also requires special care, as the dosage they receive has to be lower that adults' and is calculated carefully depending on their age and size. Some of the children had to be awakened to take their medicine and getting a child who is half asleep to swallow tablets isn't easy.

Anyone who has had children will know how quickly their condition can change. There was one boy who had been admitted during the day with a severe attack of asthma and I was told that if this recurred I should call Night Sister, who would then see if it was necessary to get a doctor. We were never allowed to call doctors ourselves, only a night sister had the authority to do so. The little boy was in a side room where I checked him regularly. He seemed sound asleep, but at around 2am I heard a loud asthmatic wheezing from his room. I called Sister Morrison, who came up immediately, but by then there was silence. He had promptly fallen back to sleep again! A couple of hours later the same thing happened, but this time I waited with him a few minutes and once again he fell back to sleep, this time for the rest of the night.

The rest of my nights passed without incident and the following week I started off as a junior again, this time on Women's Medical. However Sister Morrison came over after tea and told me to go to Women's Surgical, as someone had just had to go off sick and they were very busy. I duly made my way over to the surgical ward and found that I was on with another third year from the set below me. As I was senior I would normally be in charge, but when she offered me the keys and said she would give me the report, I stopped her.

'This is silly, me taking over at this time of night' I said. 'You've been running the ward all week and know just where you are with everything. There's only a couple of hours left so you might as well carry on and I'll be junior.'

In reality I just felt too tired to have to learn a whole ward-full of patients at that time of the morning. That was what I found most difficult about being in the pool—never really getting to know your patients and struggling to remember everything every time you changed wards. That morning I had a strange look from Night Sister when she came to do her round, but no one said anything. Nursing was a very hierarchical profession and most nurses liked to exert their hard earned seniority. It is probably the same today. Later in the week I did have to work there as senior once again.

Christmas was now fast approaching, my third since starting

nursing, and a week or so before the hospital held its annual Christmas Ball.

'We should go,' Hilary had said a few weeks earlier. 'None of us have ever been before and this may be our last opportunity.'

'I haven't got anyone to go with at the moment,' I said, 'but we could go as a group.'

'Yes, you don't have to have a partner. It could still be fun and there'll be some of the doctors there. They don't all have wives.'

We all decided to go, but my next problem was what to wear. A ball dress would be expensive, but I had recently been a bridesmaid at my cousin's wedding where I wore a long turquoise blue silk sleeveless dress. It didn't look too bridesmaidy, but to make it more suitable I bought some black lace material and made a top with three quarter length sleeves to go over it. I thought the final result looked good.

We all managed to get the time off and on the night Hilary and I both set off with all of us, plus a couple of others, split between our two cars. We had a wonderful time. I danced quite a lot, mainly with Doctor Pindar, one of the surgical housemen who I had often fed with omelettes in the ward kitchen when I had been doing nights on Men's Surgical.

My final week in the pool was back on days again, and included Christmas day itself. I started the week off on Men's Surgical, and one morning Matron came up to speak to me when she did her rounds.

'As you know, everyone is on duty on Christmas day, so nowhere is likely to be short of staff, so it's been decided that all of you in the pool can choose where you want to work that day. That is as long as you don't all want the same place. Do you know where you would like to go?'

For a moment I had hoped we might get the day off, but no such luck. However I didn't hesitate for long.

'I'd like to stay here, on Men's Surgical please.'

So that was where I spent the final Christmas of my training. Shortly after coming on duty on Christmas morning I bumped into Sister Lamb in the corridor on her way to her ward.

'I thought you were in the pool,' she said. 'Didn't you have a choice where to go today?'

'Yes,' I nodded.

'Why didn't you come and work here?' she indicated towards Women's Surgical.

I didn't know what to say, so mumbled something about already being on Men's Surgical. I was really just surprised she even remembered that I was in the pool.

The day went well, enjoyed by both patients and staff. It followed the usual routine with one of the surgeons coming in to carve the turkey. There was one young man whose injuries following a road accident had included a broken jaw, which he had to have wired. During the time it was wired he had, of course, to have a liquid diet. Now the wire had been removed, just in time for Christmas. As he had been on liquids for so long he would normally have had solid food reintroduced gradually, but he was determined not to miss his Christmas lunch. Eventually he persuaded us to let him have some, which he ate with relish. Needless to say it was all returned shortly afterwards, but for him it had been worth it, he had enjoyed it so much.

18.

Finals

January 1966; we had completed three years training—and more exams were looming. First were the hospital finals, a practical exam where we had to prepared for and carried out some procedure on the wards and were assessed by one of the sister tutors. At the same time there was a junior nurse with us and we had to explain to them everything we were doing. In my first year I had been the junior to someone taking their finals and at the time I had thought I would never be able to do all that, but now my turn had come. I did my practical on Men's Surgical, where my task was to do a dressing and remove some stitches. I was pleased with this as it was something I was quite used to doing, so it should be quite straightforward. Even so there was a lot to remember; explaining what I was going to do to the patient as well as to the junior, but it all seemed to go smoothly enough.

We all passed the exam and were awarded our black belts, just one step below a staff nurse, which meant that we were now qualified for our hospital badges. These would be awarded to us later in the year, with our hospital certificate, at the annual prize giving ceremony. So we now had just one last hurdle to cross, our State Final Exam, which we would sit in February. But sadly Hilary would not be with us. Because of the time she had been off sick she hadn't completed the necessary number of days training to qualify and she would have to wait another four months before for the next exam. It must have been so frustrating for her. After being off with glandular fever she had still had a couple of days in hand, but had been off again with a feverish cold in the autumn. After this she had been two days short, but

Matron had told her she would turn a blind eye to this, provided she had no more time off. Unfortunately she had soon been unwell again and struggled hard to keep going before having to give in. I wondered if she had come back to work too soon after her glandular fever and her immune system hadn't completely recovered, because she seemed to be getting every bug that was going around. However she had passed her hospital finals and was now working in the operating theatre, where she was soon to all intents and purposes treated as a staff nurse.

In the meantime I was working in casualty and outpatients, which were run together. Casualty consisted of an area where patients were received, a few cubicles and a treatment room, where minor procedures such as suturing and applying plaster of Paris casts to broken limbs were carried out. The outpatient section was rather bigger, with several consulting rooms and a large general waiting area. As students we were expected to help in the outpatient clinics when they were busy, so the only times we could be certain of being in casualty were weekends and evenings.

On my first morning there I was sent off to clean the hand basins and generally tidy up. There were a lot of hand basins as there was one in every consulting room to start with, and this turned out to be my job most mornings since I was often the only student on. I admit I did feel rather resentful; after all I was virtually a qualified nurse and it seemed a waste of all that training if I was doing just the work of a cleaner. On the other hand there wasn't usually much to do first thing, so at least it kept me occupied. It did, however, lead to my first run in with Staff Nurse Struthers.

I had been told to clean all the hand basins in both casualty and outpatient, but not to go into the X-ray department, which was at the back of the building adjoining outpatients. One morning after I had been there about a week I was working in one of the clinics when Staff Nurse Struthers appeared and yelled at me across the waiting room to come back to casualty. Once there she continued to berate me for not doing my job and leaving filthy trolleys lying about. I looked at her blankly as I hadn't seen any dirty trolleys, and I would certainly have cleaned them if I had. It turned out that I'd missed a room, situated opposite one of the X-ray rooms and which I had thought was part of that department. As no one had ever shown me around when I started there I thought it was not an unreasonable mistake, so I was probably not as apologetic as I should have been, especially as I was annoyed at her attitude.

A few days later I was on with her again one morning in casualty and she sent me plus another student, off to first coffee. On our return as we went in through the door we found her waiting, furious, accusing us of being late and making everyone else have to wait for their break. We were both completely taken aback as we hadn't realised we were late, but when we looked at the clock it was 9.31. So we were late—by one minute—but I still felt this was a gross overreaction. It certainly hadn't been intentional and could well have been due to a slight discrepancy between the clocks there and in the dining room.

I'd never been treated like that before in my training, even as a junior. Even Sister Lamb had never been as bad and at least when she berated you it was always out of an overriding concern for the patients. I vowed I would never behave like that as a staff nurse – or as a sister if ever I got that far. I don't believe any of us ever really deliberately did things wrong, but all of us make mistakes at times, and mistakes are more often than not at least in part due to not having things adequately explained in the first place by those in charge. I don't know whether Staff Nurse Struthers was often like that, or whether she had just taken a particular

141

dislike to me, but I never had problems with anybody else there. At other times when we weren't busy and we were all just waiting for something to happen, she could be quite amusing, regaling us with anecdotes of past incidents that had occurred in the department.

Clinics took up a lot of my time. My job was to call in patients after they arrived, weigh them and take their urine sample, which they should have brought with them. They then went back out to wait. I tested their sample and filled the results in their notes, which then went at the bottom of the pile waiting for the doctor. I was never able to go in with any of the doctors. If a patient needed chaperoning, the staff nurse on for that clinic would go in. It was all very simple and routine work which I felt could have easily been done by an auxiliary, but perhaps it was cheaper to use students.

Some clinics were very busy and the worst was Dr Horton's, one of the medical consultants who I remembered from my time on the medical wards. Morning clinics were supposed to run from 9am till 12.30pm, with another clinic starting at 2 pm. Dr Horton's clinic always went on to at least 3pm, overlapping with the afternoon session. I felt strongly that something should be done about waiting times, but the only concern everyone had was that doctors should never be held up. Everything was organized around this premise. Of course their time was valuable and they were under enough pressure as it was, but patients should be considered as well.

Everything took so long because patients would wait for an hour or so before being called in for a doctor. He would look at their notes and then decide they needed an x-ray or ECG (electrocardiogram), or both. So they were shown to the relevant department and had to wait for another hour or so. Then back to the waiting room for yet another long wait before the doctor was ready for them again. Surely patients could have gone to X-ray or ECG first, before seeing the doctor? The radiographers were usually hanging around with nothing to do until the clinic got going, after which they were rushed off their feet, so it would have been a great help to them if they could have spread the work load a bit better. But all request forms had to be signed by a doctor, even though it was obvious that someone referred by their GP for a chest problem was going to have to have a chest X-ray or if they had a suspected heart problem they would need an ECG. It was going to have to wait for more than a couple of decades before targets made managers begin to get to grips with the problem and find it could be largely resolved. Many people today complain about the targets of today's NHS, and certainly they have been grossly over used, but those of us who remember how it used to be realise the extent to which they have transformed most clinic waiting times at least.

Another problem often encountered was finding patients' notes. Those for clinics were prepared by the clerks, but some still went astray. In casualty, if a patient was admitted who had been in before, they would also have old notes that needed finding. During weekdays there was someone in the records department, where all patients' notes were stored, to look them out for us, but during evenings and weekends it was up to us. I must have spent hours hunting through shelves with thousands of notes. They were supposed to be arranged alphabetically, and cards left in place if notes were taken, but the system didn't always work.

Casualty was generally more interesting. Most of the work was treating cuts that needed suturing and fractures that needed splinting or plastering. For cuts the patients were often told to come back in a day or two to have their wound redressed and again later to have stitches removed and I enjoyed this work. They would also come back when plaster casts were ready to be removed. Sister showed me how this was done using an electric saw and I was glad it was something I never had to do. I would have been terrified of injuring the patient.

In the evenings there were the inevitable number of drunks admitted, usually after falling and injuring themselves. You soon got used to being sworn at, also to be careful since they could hit out at you, unaware of what they were doing. I never experienced any deliberate violence, but it was much less of a problem than it is today. If we got into any real difficulties we could always call on a porter to help. I also got to know some of the ambulance men and police, who frequently came in with patients, especially following road accidents.

Then there were the overdoses. Once it was established what they had taken they would have their stomachs washed out—not pleasant. It involves passing a large tube through the mouth and down to their stomach. Then water is poured into a funnel attached to the tube and when most of the water has passed through the funnel it is inverted over a bucket to siphon the water and stomach contents back. This is repeated a few times. Once done they would be transferred to a medical ward.

During training I had covered all the specialities at our hospital except the operating theatres, which I was a bit sorry about, although I think I would always have preferred ward work. Casualty was my final placement as a student, and with finals looming we had to come to a decision as to what we were going to do after we qualified.

'I think I'll do midwifery,' said Pat. 'If you want to get on in nursing it seems you really have to do at least Part 1.'

Midwifery training was then in two parts for qualified nurses. Part 1 lasted six months and covered all the theory. Part 2 was another six months and three of these (sometimes the whole six) were spent out of hospital working with a district midwife. There were few opportunities for anyone other than qualified nurses to become midwives then.

'I think if I did midwifery I would like to do the whole thing,' I said. 'Of course I would have to see how I got on, but I would like to feel I was fully qualified.'

Nancy looked doubtful. 'I'm not sure I want to do it at all,' she said. 'But at the moment I can only think of finishing here, and finals. After that I don't want to think about any more training or exams for ages.'

We all agreed about that and in the end all three of us decided we would like to get some experience as staff nurses before moving on. It was automatically assumed that you would stay on unless you gave in your notice. For finals we were joined by the set that had started three months before us. This was because there were four sets a year starting at three month intervals, but only three State Exams at four month intervals. So for our final study block we had all joined together.

'Mary Pryce is going to Staff on Women's Surgical,' Pat informed us one evening after a day in the classroom. Mary was in the set we joined with.

'She knows that already?' I was surprised.

'Yes, she was asked a while ago. I think Sister Lamb wanted her. She always gets the gold medallists, and Mary is sure to get it for our year.' Every year this medal was awarded to the best overall student, for both theoretical and practical work, and Pat was right, it was sure to go to Mary.

The final exam involved both a written and a practical component. The written papers were first. I found I was able to answer all the questions and afterwards everyone seemed to think it had gone reasonably well. The practical was a week or so later and to take it we all had to go to another hospital in Exeter. We took it in pairs, and I was with someone from the other set, who I didn't know very well. We were shown into a large classroom where all the equipment and instruments needed for just about every nursing procedure were laid out. Our task was to prepare for the admission of an unconscious patient who was suspected of taking an overdose. This was all quite straightforward, basically having such things as an airway at hand and preparing for a stomach washout, although it took a bit of time as we had to find everything. The examiners then took each of us separately and asked us some questions, none of which I can remember now. They were both very nice to us and it seemed to have gone alright, but of course you never quite knew.

We now had some six weeks to wait for our results and the question we were all wondering was where we were going to work, assuming we were all about to become staff nurses. Only two from the other set who were taking their finals with us were planning to stay on. The others had already left.

When I really thought about it there were only two wards where I wanted to work, Children's or Men's Surgical. I didn't think I had much chance of Children's, and if I wanted to specialize in that area I would really need to do my children's nurse training, which would take over another year. However Jill Merrifield on Men's Surgical kept her word and one day she told me she had just given in her notice. So there would be a vacancy there on nights. The following morning I went along to Matron's office to put in my request, which was duly granted. A couple of weeks later I started on Men's Surgical. All three of us were now on nights, Pat on Men's Medical and Nancy on Women's Surgical.

The day the results were due out arrived at last. I think I was more nervous than I had been for the exam itself and I hardly slept at all the night before they were due. I had nights off at the time and had come back from home the night before. We had to go to Matron's office in the morning at 7.30, by which time the post would have arrived, to collect our results.

We had all passed; all of us in both sets. A few nights later rather self-consciously I donned the coveted staff nurse's blue dress for the first time. We kept our black belts and as soon as I could I went in search of a nurses' silver buckle, eventually finding a lovely one in an antique shop in Exeter; rather expensive, but worth it.

Although now qualified, we had to wait until early summer for the annual presentation of hospital certificates and badges. Several of those who had left came back for the occasion and it was good to catch up with what they were doing. As expected, Mary Pryce got the gold medal for our year, plus another couple of prizes for being the best performing student in certain subjects, based on our exam performance, but to my amazement I got the prize for orthopaedics. For this I had some money to buy books, so I bought two, one on midwifery to prepare me for the future course, and the other was on art, quite unrelated to work.

19.

Qualified

Here I was, a qualified nurse at last, in my Staff Nurse's uniform on Men's Surgical. Sister Morrison must have been delighted, three more staff nurses on night duty. Nancy, on Women's Surgical, worked opposite me. We worked eight nights on and six off, always starting and finishing on a Wednesday, so we overlapped just that one night. This meant that the surgical wing was always covered by a qualified nurse. Pat, on Men's Medical, worked the same rota as Nancy, so I saw relatively little of her. Hilary was now permanently in the operating theatres, still waiting to take her finals. In theatre they had their own rota and staff there had to be on call to cover nights, so she was around some nights as well.

Much of my work was the same as I had been used to when I had worked there as a third year student, but soon I found that I was expected to take on other duties. When Nancy was off I took over checking drugs for the student on Women's Surgical, which meant Night Sister could leave her rounds there until a bit later. If the student there was worried about anything during the night she would usually come to me first. Sometimes I could sort things, if it was just, say, someone needing a painkilling injection, but if not I would tell her to call Night Sister. I still never called a doctor myself; that always had to go through one of the night sisters.

One of the first things Sister Morrison taught me to do was to how to take blood samples. This wasn't a job routinely carried out by nurses, but there were often samples that needed to be taken at 6 am, usually for measuring fasting blood sugar levels. It would normally be a job for a junior doctor, but we all knew the horrendously long hours they worked then. As well as working a full day they would often continue late into the evening, be on call over night and still have to work the next day. At least they could sleep a bit later in the mornings if we did this job for them. The blood samples were mainly needed on the medical wards, so I would have to go over there in the mornings to take them.

The next task I was taught was how to pack blood cells to be used for transfusion. In this procedure some of the liquid plasma is removed so that the blood cells are more concentrated. It reduces the volume of fluid given to a patient and so prevents the likelihood of overloading their circulation when it is used to treat conditions such as severe anaemia. Normally packed cells were prepared by a lab technician, but at night it would mean the expense of calling someone in specially, hence it was done by us. I never liked having to go to the Path Lab at night. It was located behind the hospital and you had to go out in the dark across a small yard, taking the key from Matron's office with you. Once inside, you first had to fumble to find the light switches. Then you hunted through the refrigerator where blood was stored for the correct bottle, which would have been cross-matched ready for the patient. I was used to doing this much as patients quite often had blood transfusions following surgery, but they would normally have whole blood. Now, if the cells needed packing, I would have to use a suction apparatus attached to a tap to suck off some of the fluid above the blood cells, which would have settled on standing in the fridge. The blood had to be kept sterile and I was terrified of contaminating it and rendering it useless. Sister Morrison showed me how to do it the first time, after which I was on my own. Luckily I didn't have to do it very often.

We had some quiet nights, but if this went on more than a couple of nights I would find myself sitting there wishing something would happen. At the same time I felt a bit guilty at these thoughts; after all I was wishing someone would get ill just to give us something interesting to do. Most nights, however, we had little, if any, time to sit down. We were never able to refuse to admit patients. When the ward was full, extra beds were lined up the centre. I don't know how many there would have to have been before we would need to turn patients away to go elsewhere. There were stories of beds nearly reaching the ward entrance, but I never saw them get that far. I think four or five were the most. But it certainly made our work more difficult, to say nothing of what it must have felt like for the patients.

The main problem with having beds down the middle of the ward was the difficulty of screening off patients. We tried to keep only those who were able to get up to the bathroom there, but they still sometimes needed treatments. When that happened we had to draw the curtains around the neighbouring beds at the side and pull portable screens across the ward to give them privacy. It was also difficult getting trolleys down to the bottom of the ward due to lack of space and it was certainly not a good situation when it came to considering the risks of cross infection. The problem would be solved, we were told, once the 'New Hospital' was finished.

One patient that upset me at the time was a man who had come in with a ruptured aortic aneurysm. The aorta is the main artery leading from the heart and a ruptured aneurysm leads to massive internal haemorrhage. Many such patients fail to survive, but sometimes surgery to repair the aorta can be carried out in time to stop the bleeding and they survive. This man had been admitted in the evening before I came on duty. As I arrived he was just being rushed to theatre. His wife was standing in the corridor looking stunned and bewildered by it all.

'I've told her to go home and we will phone her when there's any news,' said Staff Nurse Peak, one of the staff nurses who worked there on days, after telling me briefly what had happened. 'We let her stay until he went to theatre, but there's nothing she can do now. He could be three or four hours in there.'

I looked at the woman. Did she really want to go home? I was sure she would rather wait here, however long it took, but when I said this to Staff Nurse Peak as we went into the office, she was adamant. 'There's nowhere for her to wait and it may be ages before there's any news.'

So the woman left. I was sure Sister Morrison would have found somewhere for her to wait during the night. She was very good in this sort of situation, but it was too late to do anything now. This sort of attitude to relatives was fairly typical then. They were thought to get in the way and there were no facilities for them at all.

About three hours later word came from theatre that their attempt to save the man had failed and he had died on the operating table. Sister Morrison came over to the ward.

'You have his wife's phone number?' she asked me.

'Yes, it's here.' It was carefully recorded in the Kardex.

'Do you feel alright about phoning her? It's something you will have to get used to doing some time.'

This was a part of the job I had always dreaded, but knew it had to be faced, so I agreed. I would call his wife.

'You could wait a bit if you like. She may be asleep by now.'

I rather doubted this, so thought it better to do it straight away. It was one of the hardest things I had ever done. She answered at the first ring, confirming my suspicion that she was waiting by the phone, and she said very little on hearing the news. I just wished there was something more I could have done.

There was another patient we had who caused quite a stir, so much so that he was even mentioned on the television news. He was Russian! Remember this was at the height of the cold war, only three years since the building of the Berlin wall and Rudolph Nureyev's defection to the West. This patient was a sailor on a Russian vessel who had developed acute appendicitis when his ship was close to the British shore. He needed emergency surgery, but they didn't have facilities for this on board the ship and it would have taken too long to get him back home. Ours was the nearest hospital so, after going through various diplomatic channels, this was where he was brought. Of course no one here spoke any Russian, but a translator had been found from somewhere. His surgery went well and he made a good recovery. His bed was towards the end of the ward next to the motor cycle boys, and, as well as learning some English, he managed to teach them a bit of Russian before his discharge.

Normally we never used agency nursing staff on the wards. The only time one was ever called upon was if a patient needed specialing, such as on the eye ward if a patient had to be watched to prevent them from rubbing their eye following surgery, or occasionally if someone on the Private ward wanted one, in which case they had to pay, of course. However we had one patient on Men's Surgical who did need specialing. Martin was a young man who worked on a farm. One day he was driving a tractor along the side of a very steep Devonian hill when it overturned onto him. He had very severe crush chest injuries and was on a respirator, and nursed in the side ward. Someone needed to be with him at all times. During the day they were managing, but there wasn't anyone to spare on nights. So the local agency was called.

The trouble was that the sort of nurses who were employed by the agency were mainly used to carrying out basic nursing in people's own homes or occasionally in nursing homes. They were certainly not used to caring for anyone acutely ill, who would today be in an intensive care unit. The first agency nurse I had on with me was a middle aged woman who realised straight away that she was out of her depth and this worried her intensely. I spent quite a while with her at the beginning of the night and told her to ring the bell if there was anything at all she was worried about, which she did. I checked at regular intervals, particularly the respirator, and continued to give Martin all his drugs as necessary. This worked well enough, although she apologised profusely every time she had to call me.

'Don't worry about it,' I tried to reassure her. 'I don't mind how often you call. It is always better to err on the side of caution, so don't hesitate to ring.'

However it still worried her and after a few nights she said she couldn't do it anymore. This was a great pity because the next agency nurse was completely different. Again she was a middle aged woman, but she just did not want to be told anything and seemed to have complete confidence that she knew what she was doing, to the extent that she was a danger. One incident involved his drugs.

As there was always a nurse present and Martin was on a lot of drugs, a tray with all of them was kept in the room with him. One night he was due some of his drugs just after I came on duty. They included one that had to be given intravenously, so I injected it into the rubber tubing of his drip in the usual way. The nurse was watching me, but I thought no more about it. At midnight he was due some different drugs, including antibiotics, all of which were to be given by intramuscular injection, not intravenously this time. By chance one of the doctors arrived on the ward to see

Martin at around a quarter to twelve and I accompanied him to the side ward. As we entered to my horror I saw the nurse with the drugs drawn up about to inject them into the drip tubing as she had seen me do earlier. I stopped her quickly.

'They're due now,' she said.

'Yes, but not intravenously. These have to be given intramuscularly.'

After that I removed the tray every night and administered all the drugs myself.

I told Sister Morrison what had happened and she spoke to Matron in the morning. But the agency didn't have anyone else either able or willing to do the job, so the same nurse carried on. Not for long though. Martin's condition was beginning to go downhill when I left for my nights off and by the time I returned he had died.

One evening after I had been there around five months Sister Granger, the sister in charge of Men's Surgical on days, took me to one side after she finished giving me the report.

'Would you like to come on days for a couple of weeks?' she asked.

'Well yes. Do you need someone on days?' I was certainly surprised. The two day staff nurses both seemed like permanent fixtures, having been there since before I started training.

'Yes. Staff Nurse Peak starts on holiday next week and now Staff Nurse Freeman has gone off sick. I don't know how long she'll be off for, but I can't manage without a staff nurse for two weeks.'

So a week later I arrived for my first day shift. It was quite a change. Now there were doctor's rounds and meals to serve as well as treatments such as dressings, which weren't routinely done on nights. I soon found I was enjoying myself. At the end of the first week, however, Sister Granger had a dilemma. She was due the weekend off. Would I be able to cope from Friday evening until mid day on Monday? She was prepared to come on duty if necessary, but the ward wasn't especially busy and we even had a couple of empty beds, so I thought I should be able to cope. There were two third year students to cover my time off during the day. So at 4.30pm on Friday off she went. I was on my own—and now the admissions started!

By Saturday morning the empty beds were filled. Over Saturday and Sunday we had a string of emergency admissions, and by Monday morning, even though I had managed to get a couple of patients transferred to another ward, there were four beds up the middle of the ward. I worked as never before trying to get everything straight before Sister Granger came back on duty.

'What on earth have you been doing?' she exclaimed as she arrived on the ward.

'Oh, they just never stopped coming in,' I said.

She laughed. 'Typical,' she said. 'They were just waiting for me to go.'

Over the next week things gradually quietened down again. There were several patients due for discharge so we were able to reduce the number up the middle, making our work much easier.

One thing I did find whilst back on days was how much better I felt. I hadn't realised how much my tiredness had built up over the months of night duty and had become so used to feeling that way that I hadn't noticed. Some people can cope with it much better than others and Sister Morrison had been on nights for years. But it was clear to me that I couldn't continue indefinitely and perhaps now was the time to look for a change. Both Pat and Nancy felt very much the same and Hilary, who had by now taken and passed her finals to become a staff nurse in theatre, really wanted to get back to ward nursing again soon. It was time for us all to move on.

'I think I would like to do my BTA cert.' " Nancy said to me on one of the nights we were both on duty.

The BTA certificate was a qualification run by the British Thoracic Association (now British Thoracic Society) which, as its name implies, gave training in the care of patients with respiratory diseases. It was normally a nine month course, but Nancy could do it in six since we had all completed three months secondment in this speciality. I was interested in this as well, but thought I would do midwifery first. I said this to Nancy.

'Yes,' she said. 'I think I will too. Pat definitely wants to do midwifery, so we may go together for Part 1.'

This is what she did, doing her BTA certificate course after Part 1 midwifery. Pat completed the full midwifery training and continued to work as a midwife. Hilary got a job working on a children's ward in Gloucester, going on to work as a district nurse and then into occupational health.

I decided on midwifery and was accepted on a course in Bristol in November. So in October I worked my final nights on Men's Surgical. It was just two months short of four years since starting out on my preliminary training. I had certainly come a long way since then. Had I really become the 'sensible and responsible' Staff Nurse that Matron had said I would at the end of my training? I hope so, but now there were fresh challenges to face.

20.

Midwifery—a new beginning

Why did I decide to train as a midwife? It certainly wasn't something I had ever even remotely considered until towards the end of my nursing training. But I had worked on a maternity ward during my nurse training, so I knew a bit about what it involved and thought I would enjoy the work, plus I liked the idea of being a practitioner in my own right.

At that time the usual route to becoming a midwife was to train first as a nurse. The training was then in two parts. Part 1 was all hospital based and during this time you covered all the theory and had to conduct at least ten deliveries. Many nurses only did Part 1, mainly because it was essential if you ever wanted to progress as a nurse to a more senior post. However to become fully qualified you had to complete Part 2, a further six months, three in hospital and the final three on the district. You had to conduct at least ten more deliveries both in hospital and on district. It always seemed a bit of a waste of time to train so many nurses in Part 1 when many never had any intention of doing Part 2. At the same time for anyone keen to become a midwife it meant a total of four years training, although there were a couple of hospitals where it was possible to do a two year complete midwifery course without doing nursing first. Today it is a three year degree course in its own right.

I decided on Bristol for my training and after interview was accepted there. Although the hospital already ran the Part 2 course, they were now starting Part I as well and I was in the first set there to take this course. Since they would now be running both parts of the training, at interview the matron made it clear that pupils were expected to do both.

However I would have to see how I got on with Part 1 before finally deciding whether or not to go on to Part 2. It was certainly going to be very different to my work on a men's surgical and accident ward.

The maternity hospital was a typical red brick Victorian building. I was told that a brand new maternity hospital was about to be built as its replacement, but of course it would not be completed during my training. I seemed to be fated to work in old hospitals as the 'New Hospital' in Torquay was still not complete when I finished working there. However this hospital was in a lovely location in Bristol, adjacent to the Downs that extended towards the suspension bridge over the river Avon, and its position so high up also meant it had extensive views over the city from the wards.

During training we were always known as pupil midwives, not students. Our uniforms were quite modern for the time; plain white dresses fitted to the waist, no belt or apron. We had enough dresses to change them regularly and would be wearing gowns over them much of the time, at least in the labour ward. Our caps were also plain white, which differentiated us from the Part 2 pupils, who wore caps with a blue band on them. There were nine of us starting together and four of us, including me, were resident. The nurses' home was immediately adjacent to the hospital, but the trouble I found was that my room looked out over the road and large roundabout. Traffic never ceased; it continued all day and night and, as the roundabout was just at the top of a steep hill, all vehicles sounded as though they were revving their engines in low gears. I was used to virtually complete silence at night and for the first three nights or so barely slept at all. Eventually I fell asleep from sheer exhaustion and soon no longer noticed the noise.

We started with a couple of weeks in the classroom. Here we covered the anatomy and physiology of reproduction, much of which was revision for us, but now going into more detail than we had in our general nurse training. We also learnt about the different stages of labour. The first stage is the time during which the cervix dilates ready to allow the baby through. The second stage is the time following full dilatation of the cervix until the baby is born, and the third stage is the delivery of the placenta (afterbirth). Then there was the mechanism of delivery, which is how a baby's head fits through the pelvis. Neither a baby's head nor the outlet of the pelvis is perfectly round, which is why the most usual and best position is when a baby comes out head first facing towards the mother's back. If it faces the other way it is not quite so easy to deliver and can cause the mother a good deal of backache during labour. We also learnt about pain relief during labour, in particular how to give gas and air. We all had to try this out on ourselves, taking a few breaths so that we knew what it felt like. It made us feel a bit light headed, but very quickly wore off.

After the first two weeks we started practical work; antenatal clinics, antenatal ward, labour ward, post natal ward and Special Care Baby Unit (SCBU), and we moved round between them all every two to three weeks. We continued to have lectures and study days at intervals throughout the six months, plus three weeks of nights later on in the course. I started off in clinics together with Jeannie, one of the other pupils. Here there were plenty of opportunities to practice palpating abdomens to assess how the baby was growing and that it was the right size for the stage of pregnancy, to determine the baby's position and, of course, listen to the foetal heart rate. To listen to the heart we had to rely entirely on a simple trumpet shaped device, the foetal stethoscope, since there were no electronic aides to help us. Also there were no scans that every mother has today during pregnancy. If we needed to actually see the baby for any reason the mother would have to have an X-ray, but these were avoided unless really essential because of the risks of exposure to radiation.

There was only one midwives' clinic each week and this was the most enjoyable for us as well as patients, since we had more time to talk to them and discuss things like how to prepare for breast feeding. For some reason the doctors were unwilling to relinquish many patients to our care, preferring to see most of them themselves. I felt they didn't trust us, which was a shame as the clinic midwives had far more experience than the junior doctors. However I enjoyed the booking clinics, where all new patients came for their first visit and we had to take their history before passing them on to a doctor for a further check. We also sat in on some of the antenatal classes.

After clinics I moved on to the antenatal ward for a couple of weeks, by which time I was gaining confidence in my skills of examining patients. Several patients were in for rest because of raised blood pressure, which can be the first sign of pre-eclampsia, a dangerous complication of pregnancy, so there were frequent blood pressure rounds to do. There was also one woman who had had a small bleed when only just six months pregnant. This is known as an antepartum haemorrhage. Bleeding during pregnancy can be a sign that the placenta is not in the right place. Normally it is attached high up in the womb, but it can attach low down at the side or even across the bottom, so obstructing the opening of the cervix. This is highly dangerous because later in pregnancy or in early labour when the cervix begins to dilate, the placenta will become detached and this, as well as cutting off oxygen to the baby, can lead to sudden and very severe bleeding. Today the position of the placenta is easily determined by a scan, but since that wasn't an option then, we had to keep her in hospital for the rest of her pregnancy.

It was just too dangerous to send her home. If she started to bleed in hospital there would be no delay in performing an emergency caesarean section. On the other hand she might still go on to deliver normally, but there was no way of telling, so we couldn't take any risks. She was in for a long stay.

One afternoon shortly after I started there I was on my own for the afternoon when one of the patients rang her bell.

'My waters have broken,' she informed me.

I checked and sure enough her bed was decidedly wet. After making her more comfortable I wasn't sure what I should do next, so I consulted the midwifery text book that lived in the office. The one danger when membranes rupture is a prolapsed cord, I learnt; a rare but serious complication. We hadn't yet covered this in our lectures, but it sounded bad as pressure on the cord would cut off oxygen to the baby. So I phoned labour ward where I spoke to Sister Jennings, the sister in charge there. They seemed to be very busy, but she sent a doctor down to check the patient. In the meantime I prepared the things needed for an internal examination, which he carried out promptly. Everything was fine and I was told they would take her on labour ward shortly, as soon as they had space. I felt glad that I had done the right thing as it was still very early in my training. Being the first set to do Part 1 they often forgot that we had little or no previous experience of midwifery.

At last I was moved to the labour ward, the part of training we all looked forward to most, if with some trepidation. A couple of the others, who had started off there, had already done their first deliveries and the rest of us were quite envious. I started at the same time as Fiona, whose room was next door to me in the nurses' home, so we were able to compare notes as we went along. But before we could get our hands on any actual deliveries we had to witness at least five normal births. As I had worked on a maternity unit during my general training I knew what to expect, but some of the others had never witnessed a birth before. Now, however, when present at a delivery I tried to concentrate more on watching exactly what the midwife was doing.

One thing we soon discovered was that there was competition for deliveries. As well as us there were Part 2 pupils and medical students, and all of us had to conduct a minimum number during training. We also had to give gas and air to at least fifteen mothers, although this could be spread over Part 2 as well. Witnessing five births was no problem and Fiona and I had both done this by the end of our third day, so now we were eager to get our hands on our first delivery. Unfortunately there was a Part 2 pupil who was short of cases and she was being given priority, so we both started off giving gas and air. This is an important role. As well as helping the mother use the gas and air correctly, you were the one giving her vital support and encouragement during the later stages of labour and delivery. During the second stage, you encouraged her to push after taking a couple of deep breaths on the gas, and telling her to stop pushing and pant at the crucial time so that the baby's head is delivered gently. The midwife supervising the delivery usually had the job of giving the ergometrine injection, which was given routinely to all mothers as soon as the baby was born. This drug makes the uterus contract strongly, which speeds up the delivery of the placenta and reduces the risk of excessive bleeding, known as a postpartum haemorrhage. The third stage of labour is the time a woman is at most risk of bleeding.

Eventually my chance came. I don't remember much about my first delivery, and the midwife who was scrubbed up with me did most of the work. It was the woman's third baby, so was very quick. The midwife put her hands over

162

mine to guide me as the head was delivered, then told me to feel to check that the cord was not around the neck. I had barely time to do this when the woman pushed hard with the next contraction and the rest of the baby shot out with a rush. There seemed to be so much to remember and, being unsure of myself, I waited to be told what to do next as I went along. I spent much of the evening afterwards going over it all in my mind so that I would be quicker next time.

The next day I had another chance, with Sister Jennings scrubbed up with me. I kept one hand over the anal pad giving support to the perineum. The other hand was kept on the baby's head as the top appeared so as to help it deliver gently during her next contraction. Once the head was out I felt to make sure the cord was not around its neck. There was no cord, so I told her to push with the next contraction. The baby rotated slightly, as it should, so that the body would be born sideways on to the mother. As she pushed I held the baby's head down until the front shoulder was through, then held it up to release the posterior shoulder, after which the rest of the body slid out easily. I glanced at the clock to note the time, but at that moment there was a sudden gush of blood from the mother. Quickly I cut the cord and someone took the baby while sister, who had already given her the routine ergometrine, felt and started to massage on the mother's abdomen to stimulate her uterus to contract more strongly. I prepared to deliver the placenta (afterbirth). Thankfully the bleeding stopped as fast as it had begun, and the placenta delivered without any further problem. She hadn't lost very much blood—we estimated about half a pint— so we were not too concerned. Afterwards Sister seemed pleased at how it had gone, especially as it had been only my second delivery. I was glad I hadn't been phased by the sudden bleed, and had managed to get on with what I needed to do without having to be told every move.

After three deliveries we no longer needed someone scrubbed up with us, although a qualified midwife was always present and she would still have to put on sterile gloves to help if the woman needed an episiotomy, a cut in the perineum to widen the outlet. I watched as I was shown how to inject local anaesthetic and, after waiting a short time for it to take effect, doing the episiotomy at the height of the next contraction. We didn't have to do episiotomies during Part 1 as it could be left for Part 2, but I thought I should learn as soon as possible and I did a couple later on during the first part of my training. Of course we always tried to avoid doing them, but they are sometimes essential. If a mother, or even more importantly a baby, is getting too tired or distressed, an episiotomy can speed up delivery significantly.

The idea that husbands might like to be present at a birth was very new then and it had only very recently been allowed. However during the first stage of labour women were in a four bedded ward and it was not considered appropriate for husbands to be around when other women were in labour as well as their own wives. Instead they had to stay in the waiting room. I felt it was a shame because they could have given their wives so much support during this time. Once women were moved into the delivery room, however, husbands could be with them, although in practice very few took up the option. If they did they were told they should go out immediately if they felt unwell as we would be too busy attending to their wife to deal with them if they fainted.

It seemed a slow process, but eventually I reached my requisite number of ten deliveries, and went on to do three or four extra by the end of the course. It had been a bit frustrating at times, especially if I had been looking after a woman for a while, but when it came to the actual delivery there was someone else needing a case, so you had to hand over to them at the last minute. You were usually compensated slightly by being able to give the gas and air instead, but it wasn't the same.

21.

Babies

The post natal ward consisted of several rooms of between four and six beds, plus a couple of side rooms. It always seemed very busy. Midwives are responsible for mothers and babies up to ten days following delivery, and longer if the midwife thinks necessary. Here they normally stayed in for just seven or eight days as there weren't enough beds for them all to stay any longer. After they went home the district midwife visited daily until their tenth day. A few were booked with the district midwife for early discharge after forty eight hours. Even this is longer than many mothers stay in hospital today, with most going home after a few hours. Anyone who had a caesarean would definitely stay the full eight days, not going home until they had had their stitches removed.

Much of the work here centred around the babies. When they were first brought in from the labour ward they would have already been weighed and examined by the midwife there. Now we gave them their first bath and got them dressed. At that time we then gave them a small glucose feed to keep up their blood sugar levels. Later on we also started giving all babies an injection of vitamin K, as babies tend to be low on this at birth and it is needed to make their blood able to clot normally so that they are not prone to bleeding.

At feed times we went round helping mothers as necessary, especially those breast feeding. We always encouraged breast feeding, but would never force anyone against their will. Those who were bottle feeding were given an injection that was supposed to prevent their breasts filling up and becoming painfully engorged, but I never thought this worked very well. Then we had to make sure they knew how to change nappies, learning how to fold the large terry towelling nappies so that they fitted properly. Later we demonstrated how to bath the babies and helped the first time mothers who had never done this before. On the seventh day all babies had their Guthrie test, which tests for a fairly rare genetic disease called phenylketonuria. If a baby is affected it is important to start them on a special diet as early as possible because otherwise the disease leads to brain damage. The test involves taking a few drops of blood from the baby's heal following a small prick. Most of us didn't like the idea that we were hurting them, but although the babies might cry a bit at first, they always settled down very quickly afterwards. Babies were put in the wards next to their mothers during the day, but went into the nursery for the night so that the mothers were not disturbed by them crying.

Sometimes we would have an unmarried mother and they would often have their baby adopted. They would be given a single room so they were not near any babies and, I sometimes wondered, to keep them away from other mothers. It was still considered shameful to give birth outside wedlock. One such young mother was Pauline Sykes. She had arranged for her baby son to be adopted and he was taken straight to the nursery after his birth, where we were to look after him. But the following day she wanted to see him, and then to have him in her room for a while. When I went into her room she was crying.

'I can't let him go,' she said. 'What can I do?'

She had hidden her pregnancy from her parents and this was why she had moved to Bristol, well away from her home. She had intended to have the baby adopted so they would never know. Now she knew she could not be parted from him, so she plucked up courage and phoned her parents. It must have been a shock for them, but the following day they were there to visit her and their new grandson. Thankfully they gave Pauline their full support, which was more than some parents would have done then, and eventually they took her and her baby back home with them.

Finally I spent two weeks on the Special Care Baby Unit (SCBU) helping to look after the babies there. Here the very small or sick babies were nursed in incubators and some were so small and fragile it took a while to get used to handling them. They often had drips attached as well as feeding tubes and oxygen fed into the incubator. The worst bit for me was when I had to give them injections as they had so little flesh on them; they seemed just skin and bone.

Most of the work was one long round of feeds. Those babies not strong enough to suck were tube fed and as they got stronger bottle feeding was gradually introduced, but they were often very slow and could not be hurried. Mothers who were breast feeding would have to express their milk and we stored it in a fridge ready to give to their baby. When it neared the time that a baby was ready to go home, the mother would come to spend more time in SCBU so she could get used to feeding her baby herself. Many babies would need to be there for several weeks and some of the nurses got very attached to them. Even so it was very satisfying when they were well enough to leave us.

On one occasion I was asked to assist with an exchange transfusion on a baby with jaundice. It is quite common for babies to become slightly jaundiced a day of two after their birth. Babies are born with an excess of red blood cells and over the first few days of life some of these break down, a process which leads to a rise in a substance called bilirubin in the blood. It is bilirubin that is responsible for making their skin yellow. Slight jaundice is not a problem, but if it gets too severe it can lead to brain damage. To avoid this happening any baby with more than very sight jaundice would have a blood test to estimate the level of bilirubin. The treatment is very simple—exposure to light. Light breaks down bilirubin and is usually enough to prevent its levels getting dangerously high. We would expose as much as possible of the baby's body to light, and nursed them naked in their cot under a bright lamp. We kept them in the ward nursery where it was warm during the treatment, which was usually completed in two or three days, and just dressed them and took them in to their mothers for feeding.

Sometimes, however, jaundice can be much more of a problem; that is when it is due to rhesus incompatibility. This happens when a mother's blood group is rhesus negative and her husband's is rhesus positive. The baby may inherit the father's blood group and be rhesus positive, and the mother then produces antibodies against the baby's blood cells. What seems to happen is that during the first pregnancy a rhesus negative mother becomes sensitized. Her first rhesus positive baby is very rarely affected, but in subsequent pregnancies, if the baby is again rhesus positive, the mother's antibodies start to destroy the baby's red blood cells. This starts before the baby is born and it may die if not treated soon enough. Labour may need to be induced early so that the baby is born before it is affected too badly, and then an exchange transfusion may be necessary. Today thankfully this condition is rarely seen, at least in developed countries, as rhesus negative mothers are given an injection to prevent any harmful antibodies from being produced, so protecting any of her future children. This treatment was to become available very soon, but in the meantime exchange transfusions were the only treatment.

The baby boy that needed the transfusion had been born the previous night. His mother already had a daughter, who of course had not been affected, but this time she had needed to be induced a couple of weeks early so that her baby could be treated as soon as possible. To assist with an exchange transfusion my job was to comfort the baby and hold him still during the procedure. At the same time I had to listen to and record his heart rate at regular intervals to make sure there was no reaction to the injected blood. It is a very slow and lengthy process. Only a very small volume of blood, usually 5 mls (a teaspoonful), is withdrawn and discarded, then 5 mls of fresh blood injected as replacement into the vein in the baby's umbilicus. This has to be done very slowly and is repeated until the doctor estimates enough has been replaced.

Once the transfusion was completed the baby was kept in SCBU for a few days and his bilirubin levels rechecked regularly in case he needed a further treatment. Luckily this wasn't needed and he was soon able to be reunited with his mother in the ward.

Generally I enjoyed the experience of working there, but at the same time I realised it was not something I would like to do for long. I found the pace of work too slow, spending most days just feeding babies. Many were slow to feed, so a lot of patience was needed, and I think it takes a special kind of nurse to undertake this sort of work. I preferred to be kept more active, so was glad when I returned to the wards once again.

22.

More babies

I enjoyed being in Bristol, finding it quite a change to be living in a large city after working in Torquay for almost four years. There was a lot of studying to do during our time off, but I found time for some relaxation. Fiona and I went to the theatre and concerts a few times and I went out with Jeannie to a couple of discos. Jeannie lived in a flat in Clifton which she shared with two others. It was on the top floor of a large crescent and looked out across the Avon Gorge. It made me think I should move out of the nurses' home, but we would all have to live in when we went on district in Part 2, so I decided it wasn't worth it.

At the end of the six months we had our Part 1 exams, which were a couple of three hour papers, We all passed our exam and all but one of us, who decided to get married instead, were going to continue our training. We had a month off before beginning Part 2, a much welcomed break, although Jeannie got a temporary job with a nursing agency to get some money to supplement her meagre pupil midwives' salary.

As one of our original set had left, we now had a new pupil joining us. I met her in the nurses' home on my return after our month off. This was Alison, a red head from Birmingham, and her presence was to liven up our group considerably. There were also a couple more sets who had started doing Part 1 by then, so the nurses' home was much busier and I got to know several of them as well. It was now June and we were in for a good summer, too good to stay in the city, so almost every other weekend some of us who were off duty would take off together to the coast. Sometimes this would only be as far as Weston-Super-Mare, which was an easy drive in my car. Other times we hitch-hiked much further, to Devon or Cornwall, staying in youth hostels.

On one occasion there were four of us and we decided to split into two pairs and see who could get to one of the youth hostels in North Devon first. I was with Alison and we got there in good time that evening, but there was no sign of the others. They never arrived, although the hostel warden kept the doors unlocked for them much later than usual. The hostels normally closed at 10 pm then. The next morning we met them waiting for us outside looking rather bedraggled. It turned out they had arrived late and didn't know what to do, so they sat in a bus shelter out of the fine drizzling rain that had started. A couple of young men had passed, and a moment later returned, asking them what they were doing. On hearing that they had nowhere to go the men looked really concerned. As they were staying in a guest house they could hardly offer to take in two young women for the night, but they then very kindly offered them their car to sleep in. So they had slept in a car all night.

Another time three of us travelled by car to St David's in Wales, only to find the hostel there was full up. Not knowing what to do we wandered into a local pub, by which time it was gone 10.30, less than half an hour to closing. In that time we had no less than three offers of accommodation. Eventually we took up the offer of someone's caravan for the night.

In the meantime our work and studies was continuing. The first three months of our Part 2 training was all in the hospital. Our studies now included more on the social and legal aspects of our work, such as when and how a birth had to be registered and when a woman qualified for maternity benefits. We had to conduct at least another ten deliveries and, although always supervised by qualified midwife, we were left to make more decisions on the management of labour ourselves. There was still competition for cases, but I managed thirteen deliveries in the end.

Women were often allowed to labour for far longer than they would be today. Drugs to speed things up were not used so readily then. It was disheartening sometimes to spend a whole day looking after someone but they were still nowhere near delivering by the time you went off duty. I also felt desperately sorry for those who were in labour when we left, only to find them still there, still not delivered and looking absolutely exhausted the following morning. I felt even more sorry for women when, after struggling through hours of a prolonged first stage, maybe even getting to the second stage of labour, and then ending up with an emergency caesarean section, perhaps for failing to progress further or if the baby became too distressed. Today many of them would have had a caesarean section much sooner, but this operation was seen then as very much a last resort, to be avoided if at all possible. Of course they were always done under a general anaesthetic then, rather than an epidural, which would usually be used today. Even so we all witnessed one or two caesareans as a midwife would always be there to take the baby. She would be handed a sterile towel, which she then held out to receive the baby from the doctor doing the operation. Today I believe the caesarean rate can be as much as one in four births in some hospitals. Many people, including myself, think this is far too high, but at the same time the neonatal death rate is significantly lower, which has to be good.

Linda Reaves was someone who I am sure would have had a caesarean today. She was expecting her first baby and I admitted her when she arrived in labour, examining her and giving her the routine enema and shave that we gave every woman then. She was getting good contractions so I needed to examine her internally to assess her progress. By now I was allowed to examine patients internally without a midwife checking and I found she was three fingers dilated. We always measured dilatation in finger widths then, which sounds rather vague as people's finger widths can vary, but in practice when double checked our assessments were usually pretty consistent. Her membranes were bulging and Barbara, the midwife with me, told me to rupture them to release the liquor, which should help to stimulate labour. This I did and dark green stained liquid was released. This liquid, the liquor as it is called, should be clear and the green discolouration was due to meconium. Before birth the baby's gut is filled with this dark green, almost black substance, and it is passed during the first couple of days following birth. Sometimes, however, if the baby is in any way distressed, they pass some before birth, so discolouring the liquor. It is not a good sign.

We informed the doctor on call, but the foetal heart rate was good, so he said to continue and let him know if there was any further change. We gave Linda some pethidine for pain and made frequent checks on the baby's heart rate. A few times it slowed slightly, but recovered quickly to the normal rate of between 140– 150 beats a minute. All seemed to be well and two or three hours later she reached the second stage and started to push. I listened in again, and now the heart rate had dropped to a hundred. We called the doctor as the baby needed to be delivered quickly and forceps might speed things up, but the head was coming down well, so I prepared for the delivery. When the doctor arrived the heart rate had dropped further and he told me to do an episiotomy quickly with the next contraction, which I did, and the baby's head was out. I felt around the neck and found the baby's cord was wound tightly twice round. It was so tight it was difficult to clamp and cut, but I managed, enabling the baby girl to be fully delivered. But she made no attempt to cry as I handed her pale limp body to Barbara, who took her over to the doctor.

The baby needed to be intubated, that is a small plastic tube inserted into her windpipe to get oxygen into her lungs, and thankfully she soon gained some colour, becoming pink and breathing on her own. Once the tube was removed from her throat she gave a few weak cries. It had been a close thing. The problem must have been due to the cord around her neck, which would have restricted blood flow to the baby causing her distress. We sent her to SCBU so she could be monitored closely for a while, but she was soon well enough to go to the post natal ward with her mother. She seemed none the worse for her experience, and I just hoped there were no long term effects from her difficult birth.

Another day when I came on duty for a late shift I was told to go and look after Dawn Mottram. It was her first pregnancy and she was already fully dilated. I went into the labour room eagerly, looking forward to the prospect of another delivery. But the midwife I joined was looking a bit dubious.

'She's been fully dilated for almost an hour and there's no progress,' she told me.

We never allowed patients to push for more than two hours in the second stage, which meant there was still another hour to go, so we might be lucky. However Dawn had been labouring since the previous evening and was exhausted, becoming quite distressed with it all. So after a few more contractions without any progress a doctor was called to do a forceps delivery. He decided to call the anaesthetist to give her a light anaesthetic during the procedure.

Once she was asleep the doctor delivered a baby boy, a bit small, but crying lustily. I wrapped him in a towel and put him in the cot, and was just preparing the label to attach to his ankle when the doctor said 'There's another one.'

There was another baby. She had undiagnosed twins. A minute later a baby girl was delivered, also in good condition. Someone found another cot and she was placed in this next to her brother. Once the doctor had finished I was left to sit with Dawn until she came round from the anaesthetic. So I was able to give her the news that she had both a son and daughter. She was delighted.

Undiagnosed twins were not all that uncommon then and these were not the only ones I came across during my time as a midwife. Today they are rare since they would be diagnosed by the scan early in pregnancy.

Then there were breech deliveries. These were normally considered a doctors province, but we all had to know what to do in case of an emergency. Although we always palpated women very carefully to determine the position of a baby before birth, a breech can sometimes be missed until the baby is almost ready to deliver. Therefore we always took the opportunity to watch when there was such a birth. The first one I witnessed was quite early in my training. The woman was placed in what is known as lithotomy position, that is with her feet held up in stirrups and her buttocks at the edge of the base of the bed. This is important for a breach delivery. I watched as the baby's buttocks appeared, and could see that it was a boy. He had his legs extended forwards in front of him, and as his body was born the doctor had to free each leg. Then the arms had to be freed carefully, after the shoulders were out. Then he let the baby hang. This sounds strange, but it helps the head rotate to the best position for its delivery. Once rotated the baby's body is raised. This is the critical stage. Once the body is out the cord is compressed and no oxygen can get to the baby, which means time is of the essence. However, the head needs to be delivered slowly. If it pops out too quickly it can cause brain damage from the sudden release of pressure. Often forceps are used to have better control, and this is what the doctor did now, plus an episiotomy to make delivery easier. The baby cried immediately and I watched the midwife take him to his cot. I noticed she had to wrap him up firmly to keep his legs down. Because he had had his legs extended up in front of him before birth, that was the position he was used to. It would take a few days to adapt to the normal position.

The three months in hospital were soon over. As well as working on the wards and attending lectures, we had to write up detailed case studies, which were to form part of our final assessment. This included three bookings we had taken and three case histories of women we had delivered ourselves. This all had to be done in our own time and the tutors checked what we had done to make sure they were all completed correctly and in the correct format before we finished our time there. I had delivered another fourteen babies and was feeling reasonably confident in my work. But now we were preparing for a big change, where we all knew we would have to begin to undertake much more responsibility, often working on our own. For the next three months we would be on the district.

23.

The District

For the next three months we were all allocated to specific districts within the city where we were to work under a district midwife. We had to live in digs within our area and these had been arranged for us. We were expected to buy bicycles to get around visiting patients, although when we were called out to someone in labour at night we could call the ambulance station, who would arrange a taxi to take us. This was needed not only because of the equipment we had to take with us, but because we could often be called some distance away to a neighbouring district covering for anyone off duty.

Although we were meant to have bicycles I decided from the outset that I would use my car.

'You won't get any petrol allowance,' everyone told me. 'So it will be entirely at your own expense.'

I realized that, but we were starting in September, so the good weather we had been enjoying couldn't last much longer and I didn't relish the thought of cycling around in the rain. Alison had also decided to use her scooter at her own expense, as it would be quicker to get around on. As luck would have it, I was to work in Bedminster, probably the most compact district of all in the city, with its rows of Victorian terraces, two up and two down. I could have walked to many of my patients. Most of the homes I was to visit had been bought by young couples and modernized by them. Some were owned by the grandparents, the young mother staying with her own mother while she got used to caring for her newborn. It was generally considered to be a good area to work, with few of the social problems sometimes encountered on the large council estates. My digs were in one of these terraced houses, with a couple and their two children, a girl of ten and a boy of two. I couldn't have lived anywhere better; they were a lovely family and made me feel so welcome.

On my first morning Sister Wilkins, the midwife to whom I had been allocated, arrived promptly at 7.45 am. She had been working on district for years and only had a couple more years to go before retiring, she told me later. Her experience showed in her work, always calm and unflappable. That first day she came in her car to collect me, as I would be doing the rounds of routine post-natal visits with her so that she could show me what to do. All the bags containing the equipment I would need for my work had been there waiting for me when I moved into my digs the evening before and I had already spent some time examining them all to see what they contained; equipment for deliveries, taking blood pressure, a foetal stethoscope, miniature oxygen cylinders for babies, miniature scales from which babies could be suspended in a nappy in order to weigh them. Today I would need just one bag; the nursing bag, which contained all I needed for post natal visits caring for new mothers and their babies.

We visited mothers twice a day for the first three days following their delivery, then daily until their tenth day, and longer if they needed more help. Some of them had given birth at home, others in hospital and had either been early discharges at forty eight hours following delivery, or sent home on their eighth day, in which case we would only be visiting them for a couple of days. Going round with Sister Wilkins I began to learn the layout of the district, important for when I would be on my own, although I was ready armed with a detailed street map. A couple of days later, once she was happy that I knew what to do, I was on my own. Every day I had my own list of visits, and I had to leave a copy of this, in the order I intended to do them, at my digs so that I could be found if anyone went into labour.

I soon began to enjoy myself, always welcomed into the families and offered endless cups of tea. Some mothers needed more help than others, especially if it was their first baby, although quite a few had the grandmother close at hand all too ready to give assistance and advice. Babies were weighed every other day and we showed the mothers how to bath them. They were usually bathed in large washing up bowls set on a low coffee table; very few had purpose made baby baths then. If it was their first baby we would stay with them when they bathed their babies for the first time, ensuring they knew how to hold them securely, as many were afraid of them slipping in the water. If all was well and the baby gaining weight we could discharge them on the tenth day into the care of a health visitor.

There were often home assessments to do as well. Anyone wanting either a home delivery or an early discharge forty eight hours after delivering in hospital had to have their home assessed to ensure it was suitable. I did a few of these visits with Sister Wilkins before doing them on my own. If I was doubtful about any I would refer them on to her.

Then there were antenatal visits for those already booked for home delivery. Sister Wilkins would join me for these where, as well as their routine antenatal examinations, we would have to make sure everything was prepared for the birth. The mattress of the bed would need protection, as would the bedroom carpet, if there was one. Newspaper should never be used because the black newsprint would get onto everything, but sheets of brown wrapping paper were ideal and the parents were expected to provide this. I had the list of all women we had booked for home delivery and we visited them every week during the last month before they were due, so I soon met them all.

We had to have a minimum of ten home deliveries during our three months on district. There had never been any problem with this in the past, with midwives back at the hospital telling us how they had conducted thirty or more during their three months. But the trend towards hospital births had begun and hence numbers of home births were dropping drastically. Virtually all first babies were now delivered in hospital and it was apparent that soon there would have to be a change in the regulations for training as it was going to be impossible for pupils to get the required number of cases. In the meantime, however, there were still enough for us. I had well over ten women booked, on my district and, even though I might miss one or two on my days off, I would get more on other districts either where there were no pupils or when I covered for their days off.

I had a socket in my room at my digs where I could plug in the phone at night so that I could be called if anyone went into labour. On my third night I was deeply asleep when it started to ring. It took me a moment to come to and realize what it was. It was Sister Simons, the midwife on a neighbouring district, to say one of her patients had started labour and her pupil was off, and she would pick me up in five minutes. I looked at my bedside clock; 2.15 am. It only took a minute to dress and I was downstairs waiting with my equipment when her car arrived.

'Pop your bags in the boot and jump in,' she said.

I did as I was told and she opened the passenger door for me.

'Tricks—in the back,' she said sharply, as I made to get in, and I saw she was speaking to a small Jack Russell , who did as it was told, jumping off the passenger seat into the back of the car. I got in and looked round at the dog, who bared its teeth at me, but stayed where it was. Tricks, I soon learnt, went everywhere with Sister Simons, waiting in—and guarding—the car while she visited patients.

Our patient tonight, Sonia Greg, was expecting her third child and had given birth to both her other two at home. She knew the procedure well. By the time we arrived she was getting strong contractions. I examined her and found her cervix was already a good four fingers dilated. Her previous child had been born only eighteen months ago, which meant this labour shouldn't take long, so we started her on gas and air. Less than an hour later her membranes ruptured and she wanted to push.

'You get yourself gloved up ready,' Sister told me. 'This one's going to be quick.'

She was right. With her next contraction we could see the top of the baby's head coming down fast, and the following contraction her baby daughter was born.

Everything went smoothly. The placenta was delivered and she didn't need any stitches. Having made her comfortable holding her new baby daughter we called up her husband, who was waiting downstairs with the grandparents. They would already have heard they baby's cries, so were waiting eagerly for the news.

There was still a lot to do. The baby needed to be weighed, then bathed and dressed and given her first feed. Mrs Greg had breast fed both of her previous children, so needed little help putting this one to the breast. It still took well over an hour to finish, so it was after 5 am before I got back to my digs. Sister Greg told me to go back to bed for a bit. She would contact Sister Wilkins and tell her I would be starting my morning rounds a bit late.

We were supposed to have a qualified midwife with us for the first five home deliveries. After that, if both we and our midwife were happy, we were on our own. However things did not always work out as planned.

My third home delivery was Maggie Breery. She was expecting her second child and had been having some irregular contractions on and off most of the night. They now seemed to be getting a bit stronger, so she called us at around 6 am. However by the time we arrived she was still only 2 fingers dilated and her contractions seemed to have fizzled out. She was tired, having been kept awake with her contractions most of the night, and now she started to doze off. Sister Wilkins and I sat quietly together with her in the darkened room. After a while Sister looked at her watch, it was nearly 7.30 am.

'She seems to be sleeping, so I'll nip back home and get a few things sorted out,' she said. 'I just need to make a couple of phone calls, so shouldn't be more than fifteen minutes or so.'

She only lived a short way away. Virtually no patients had phones then so she couldn't call from there. After she left I continued to sit with Mrs Greg and about ten minutes had elapsed when suddenly she opened her eyes.

'I want to push,' she said urgently.

I put the light on and looked. She was fully dilated, the top of the baby's head clearly visible. I made for the bedroom door thinking I could get her husband to go and call Sister Wilkins, if she wasn't already on her way back. But I didn't get very far.

'It's coming, it's coming!'

I just had time to open the delivery pack and put on my gloves before catching her baby.

Everything went well and two or three minutes later, after delivering the placenta and having a quick tidy up, I called her husband to meet his new son. He hadn't been there long when there was a knock on the door—Sister Wilkins—and he went down to let her in.

'It's a boy.' I heard him say.

Sister came pounding up the stairs. Once she was over the shock she checked everything I had done and seemed happy with it all.

After my fifth delivery I was considered safe to be on my own. The procedure now was that once the patient was fully dilated I should send the husband, or any other member of the family who was there, out to call Sister, so that she would be on her way there to help if anything untoward occurred. We had to make sure every husband had a good supply of sixpences, the coin then taken by call boxes. Several of my deliveries were in neighbouring districts to my own and when called to these at night I stopped using my car and used the taxi provided by the ambulance service. This was mainly because it could be quite difficult to find the way in a strange area in the dark, especially as house numbers are often difficult to see. In my own district, where I knew where I was going, I still used my car.

I felt pretty confident in my work, although we always had to be prepared for the unexpected. There were two main complications we dreaded. One was that the baby did not breathe properly after delivery. We carried a drug we could inject to stimulate breathing as well as small oxygen cylinders. The other was that the mother had a serious bleed and in this case we could call what was known as the Flying Squad. This was based at Southmead hospital, a large maternity hospital, and they would send an ambulance with both an obstetrician and midwife to help with the emergency. Luckily I never had anything like this happen to me, but one of Alison's patients did have a still birth. Thankfully for her the midwife was also present at that delivery, so she could in no way be blamed.

Some husbands would stay to be present at the birth. As I have said, this was quite a new idea then. I would always ask if they wanted to be there. Some would give an emphatic 'no', but most would say they were not sure. I took this to mean that they would like to be present, but were apprehensive at the thought. So I started by encouraging them to be with their wives and giving them support during the first stage of labour. Then they could leave at any time when it came to the actual birth. None of them ever left and all found it an amazing experience. I remember one husband who had sustained a back injury a few days earlier. It was too painful for him to sit with his wife, so he lay down beside her on the other side of the bed. When it came to the birth he wasn't able to get up, so he stayed where he was. I don't think he could really see very much of the birth from his position.

Sylvia Newland was another lady I delivered. It was her third baby and everything went well, but on the fourth day following the birth both she and her husband were looking worried when I arrived for my morning visit. She did not look well.

'The baby is fine, but she's been up all night with terrible indigestion,' her husband told me looking at his wife. 'She's tried all sorts of indigestion medicine, but none makes any difference at all. She's never had it before."

Alarm bells immediately rang in my mind. Sometimes what feels like indigestion can really be due to pain in the chest; it is a sort of referred pain. Sister Wilkins was on her days off or I would have called her first, so as it was I called her GP, who said he would visit. I went on with my visits, but went back later. I had been right. She had been admitted to hospital diagnosed as having had a pulmonary embolism. This is when a blood clot has formed in a vein, usually in the leg, known as deep vein thrombosis, or DVT. A bit of the clot then can break off and go to the lungs, with potentially serious consequences. Blood clotting in the leg veins is a well known complication following any period of inactivity, such as after surgery or long-haul air travel. Today all patients in hospital are given anti-DVT socks to wear as a preventative measure.

Luckily for her it must have been a small clot and after treatment Mrs Newland made a complete recovery. It wasn't long before she was home again. In the meantime while she was in hospital, her baby remained at home, so we had to visit regularly to make sure her husband was coping.

One day I had just got back to my digs for lunch when I received a phone call to say a woman in premature labour was giving birth in an ambulance in the road very close by. They called me because I was the nearest. I was there within a couple of minutes to find the ambulance men had already delivered the baby. Now the mother was sitting up holding the tiny baby boy. But when I looked at him I could see his colour was not good. I took him from his mother. He was barely breathing, so I started to give him oxygen. Apparently the baby had cried well immediately after he was born, but now he was just giving irregular gasps. This often happens with premature babies—they cry immediately after they are delivered, but don't have the strength to continue after that. I stayed with them in the ambulance as we continued the journey to hospital and the ambulance men called ahead to let them know about the baby. They had an incubator ready when we arrived, so I handed over to them. Sadly the baby, who had been born two months early, died the following day.

During my three months on district I conducted fourteen deliveries, well over the requisite ten. But I could see the trend towards hospital births was unstoppable. My feelings towards this were mixed. Women always seemed far more relaxed in their own familiar surroundings than they were in hospital and I felt you couldn't beat home for a straightforward normal birth. Of course I was lucky in that everything went well with all my cases, but things will occasionally go wrong, so there is no doubt that hospital is safer for both mother and baby. I was glad I had this experience on district and felt I had trained just in time. If it had been only a couple of years later it would have been very different with the dwindling numbers of home births. I loved the work and wondered about whether I should see if I could continue after qualifying if there was a vacancy, but you are very much on your own in the community, so I thought I should really get a bit more experience first. Even so I think I was sure even then that it was the sort of work I would want to return to one day. But before I could think about that I had to pass the final exam.

24.

Exam chaos

During our time on district we had still to attend some lectures, and to write up three more detailed case studies of women we delivered at home, plus another three bookings made for home deliveries. All these were entered together with those from our time at the hospital in a special book provided and had to be submitted as part of our final exam, which was a practical. Our examiners there would have seen the book and could ask us questions on it.

The exam was a week after we finished on district and several of the others went away during this time, but because I had been off sick with tonsillitis during my three months at the hospital, I had to go back there to make up the few days I'd missed. My exam was then only a couple of days later, so I stayed on in the Nurses' Home.

The day of our exam finally arrived. I was well prepared, going to bed in good time the night before so that I would be fresh in the morning to drive the few miles to Southmead Hospital, where the exam was to be held. The exams were due to start at 9 am and my twenty minute slot was at 9.30 am. I got out of bed a few minutes after the alarm went off, crossed the room and opened the curtains—and stared in horror. Everywhere was covered in around six inches of snow!

I tried to think what to do. I had never driven in snow before, so perhaps I should go by bus. But at that point I realised there was an eyrie silence outside. There was hardly any traffic at all; of course it would not be able to get up the steep hill to the Downs. So my only option was driving. I set off as soon as I could, driving extremely slowly. There was very little other traffic and everything was fine until I came to a slight hill, which was completely blocked by sliding vehicles. I turned around to try a different route, and soon got to a back entrance to the grounds of Southmead Hospital. But immediately inside there was a steep slope up, and here the car went slower and slower, wheels spinning, and stopped about two thirds of the way. I backed to the side wondering what to do when a man approached.

'You can't stop here,' he said. 'Ambulances have to get by.'

'I know,' I replied, 'but I can't get any further, and I have to take an exam here this morning.'

At that point a couple more men appeared and together they pushed me the rest of the way up the slope. Once on level ground I made my way to the midwifery school and parked there without any difficulty.

It was just coming up to 9 am, so I was in very good time. There were four other candidates in the changing room, none of whom I knew, so I started to get into my uniform ready. At that moment one of the tutors who was organising it all appeared.

'Alright everyone, we must get started,' She signalled to me. 'Quickly – get ready.'

'But my exam isn't until 9.30,' I said.

'That doesn't matter. Not everyone is here yet, so you can go in now.'

We were due to go into the exam in batches of half a dozen of us at a time and each candidate would be randomly assigned a patient to examine. Clearly not all candidates had arrived, so I was to go in now to make up the numbers.

There was no time to feel nervous. I rapidly pinned on my cap and followed the group. The first four were all shown into one large room with four curtained off bays, each with a patient they were to examine. I was taken to another room off to the side, again with four bays. Here I was shown into one of them and met my patient. I had ten minutes to take her history and examine her, after which I would have a further ten minutes to present my findings to two examiners, who would then question me together. The whole thing would take twenty minutes.

I got on with what I was supposed to do and on palpation I found my lady, a young woman with her first pregnancy, was expecting twins. It was all straightforward and I was soon finished and ready for the examiners, but none appeared, so we just chatted while waiting. Eventually a small dark haired woman looked in.

'Are you waiting to be examined?' she asked.

I confirmed that I was.

'Well we had better get on. I'm afraid there's only me'

I did my presentation of the patient I had examined, after which the examiner began to ask me some questions. But we didn't seem to have got very far when the bell rang to signal the end of the allotted time. It was over.

Going back to the changing room the extent of disruption caused by the snow was now apparent. It wasn't just candidates who were delayed, but also the examiners—hence there had only been one available to examine me. It turned out that trains were unable to get into Temple Meads station and passengers had to get off outside it and walk along the track. Then there was the problem of getting to Southmead with virtually no buses able to get up the steep hill from the city centre. The tutors were doing a sterling job answering frantic calls from exam candidates who were held up, assuring them that they would be able to take the exam when they arrived, however late they were.

When I got back to the changing room I found Alison had just turned up looking both shaken and flustered.

'I fell off my bike,' she said. 'A very kind gentleman helped me up. He said I shouldn't be riding a scooter in these conditions and asked me where I was going. When I told him it was the hospital he said I was going the right way about it!'

She didn't have any time to recover as the tutor appeared and said she was to go in next. I waited for her to finish. When she came out it was clear things had not gone well.

'I just couldn't think straight. I really messed up and know I've failed. I wouldn't have passed myself on that!'

While she had been in there two more of our set arrived together, followed very shortly after by Jeannie. Like the rest of us they had had a difficult journey, even though they didn't have all that far to come.

'I don't know how we are going to get back, but we'll think of that later,' Jeannie said.

'I can give you lift,' I said. 'I'm in no hurry.'

In the end I gave them all a lift back, with Alison following behind on her scooter. They were all very grateful, but in reality I had an ulterior motive. If I got stuck in the snow they would be able to push. However we had no problems on the journey and Alison and I spent most of the rest of the day with Jeannie at her flat.

I stayed on in Bristol for a couple more days until the snow had melted before going home for a prolonged Christmas break. We didn't have to wait long for the results; I had passed. Sadly Alison had been right, she failed. I felt she had been extremely unfortunate as she hadn't had time to recover from her journey to Southmead before being rushed into the exam. She would have to wait until the spring before she could retake, so she decided to fill in the time by going back to the maternity hospital to take their three month course in the care of premature babies.

As far as I know nobody in the set I qualified with went on to practice as a midwife. They all said they wanted to get back to general nursing. Jeannie went back to the agency working on a men's medical ward and Fiona got a night sister's post in a general hospital. After she finished her course and passing the exam at her second attempt Alison went abroad. One of the other married pupils went on to do what we often referred to as Part 3—that is she had her own baby—and I lost contact with the others. It seemed a waste of all the training not to use it, but this was quite common. Many nurses trained simply to get the qualification as it was good for their CV and often required if you wanted to progress in your career to a more senior posts.

25.

First steps as a qualified midwife

Now I had to do something about getting a job. I was fed up with never having any money after being on a pupil midwives' salary for so long, so decided to join a nursing agency where I would earn more than if I was employed directly by a hospital. I worked for a few weeks on a ward in a nearby hospital for patients with respiratory diseases, but I think I always wanted to get back to midwifery, so the agency found me a job as a staff midwife on a small maternity unit not far from Bristol. The unit was for patients either under their GPs or under the hospital consultant, about half and half. It wasn't a training school and I was glad not to have any pupils. I felt I needed the experience of working as a qualified midwife before having to supervise pupils myself.

I soon came to enjoy the work there. Sister Jarrett ran the unit and treated us all as professionals. In the morning there was a list of all the routine jobs, including things like any four hourly observations of TPRs and blood pressures, checking and restocking equipment in the labour rooms and making up feeds for the babies. There were no readymade feeds available then and I quite enjoyed that job, working quietly in a tiny kitchen, measuring out and mixing the powdered milk with boiling water and pouring it into freshly sterilized bottles. We were left to organize what we did each day amongst ourselves and tick things off the list as we went along. It was also up to us when we took our coffee and meal breaks. We were trusted to see that there was always cover left on the ward and we just had to pop our heads round the office door to let her know when we were going.

The unit was all run as one, which meant we were able to care for women right the way through their stay, from when they were first admitted, through labour and delivery, and afterwards until their discharge home. I got good all round experience because, with half of them booked by their GPs, we had plenty of normal births. For these cases we had to call their GP when the delivery was imminent so that they could get there in time. The GPs always wanted to be present, even though they usually had nothing to do, just occasionally some suturing. The main reason for this was that they were able to claim an additional fee if they were present at a birth. On one occasion I didn't call in time and the GP wasn't too pleased!

There were a couple of junior sisters on the ward and they kept a bit of an eye on me at first, until they were sure I was competent. One of the first few women I admitted in labour was Jane Grimond, expecting her second child. She was in strong labour when she came in one afternoon. I was on with Sister Grey, who helped me get her into the labour room. I palpated her abdomen and everything felt normal, with what is known as a cephalic presentation, which means head first. She was already getting some urge to push so I did an internal examination. I found her cervix was a good four fingers dilated, showing she was well on in labour, but now I was confused. Normally through the opening of the cervix we feel the hard bones of the baby's skull, but what I felt was completely different. I could feel a limb and behind it something soft that I thought must be the baby's buttocks. It must be a breech presentation. Could I have missed that on palpation? We always feel very carefully to make sure we don't miss a breech presentation. If it is a breech it is usually possible to feel the hard head of the baby high up, just beneath the mother's ribs

'What's the matter?' Sister Grey asked, as I must have looked confused.

'I'm not sure. It may be a breech,' I replied.

'That's not a breech,' she said, quickly checking the abdomen.

At that moment, as I was feeling what I thought was a leg, it got hold of my finger – and it all became clear.

'It's a hand,' I said. 'The baby has got hold of my finger. It's a face presentation and it's got its hand in front of its face.'

What I had first thought was the baby's bottom was a face and I had been feeling the cheeks.

'Which way round is it?'

This was important. I quickly went over in my mind what I had been taught about delivering a baby with a face presentation, as it is quite rare and I had never witnessed one during training. With a face presentation the baby's head is flexed backwards rather than forward as is usual and it can only deliver normally if the chin is facing forward towards the front of the mother. If it is facing back delivery is impossible to fit through the mother's pelvis and she would need a caesarean. Luckily it was the right way round. Even so this position doesn't fit all that well through the birth canal and she would undoubtedly need an episiotomy to help it through. Her labour was progressing fast and she was soon delivered successfully with a baby boy. His face was a bit puffy and bruised, which is as expected being born this way, and we had to reassure his mother that this would soon clear. It took a couple of days, but at last she felt confident to show off her beautiful baby boy. This was the only time I delivered a baby with a face presentation during all my years as a midwife.

Here the husbands were not encouraged to stay with their wives during labour and delivery. They were sent home and told to ring later. On one occasion I answered the phone to someone enquiring about his wife. As I hadn't delivered her myself I asked the sister who was on with me what she had had. She looked at me in surprise.

'But I only just spoke to her husband and told him,' she said. 'So who's that?'

In fact we couldn't be sure which of the calls was from her husband so, in case this one was the genuine father, I had to give him the news as well.

Another time we had a husband who, after he rang and had been given the good news of the birth of his son, went out to celebrate. After he had had a few pints he decided to ring us again, and continued to do this repeatedly about every ten minutes or so. We were quite busy that evening, so eventually I called the switchboard and got them to stop putting through any more calls from him.

Another woman I remember was Lynda Blake. She was thirty eight weeks pregnant when she came in having had a sudden severe pain, which she wasn't sure was a contraction. When I palpated her I found her uterus quite tense making it difficult to feel the baby's position. I tried to listen to the baby's heart, but couldn't hear anything. With no electronic aids to help us we had to rely entirely on the foetal stethoscope. However I persisted, trying in different positions and after a few moments to my relief I could just hear a faint beat.

The sudden pain followed by a tense and tender uterus could be a sign that she had suffered an internal bleed. Sometimes the placenta can start to detach itself, causing bleeding within the uterus. As the placenta is responsible for supplying oxygen to the baby, this is a serious complication. The doctor came to examine her.

'There's no foetal heart,' he said to us after he finished. He looked at her notes. 'But it says here that you heard it when she came in.' He looked at me.

'Yes. It was very difficult. It was very faint.'

He continued to ponder over her notes. Then he looked up.

'Well, I don't want to do a caesarean on a dead baby, but if you heard something it may still be alive and we will have to do it.'

I got her ready and, together with a porter, took her down to theatre. Once she was anaesthetized I went into theatre with her to take the baby when it was delivered. By now I was decidedly nervous. I was the only one who had heard the foetal heart. Could I have been mistaken? Sometimes when you listen you can hear the mother's pulse beating instead, but the baby's heart rate is much faster, around 140 beats a minute, so it is usually easy to distinguish between the two. Another possibility of course was that the baby had died since I listened. Even so they were only doing the operation because of me and a caesarean wasn't something undertaken lightly then—it was considered quite a major operation—so I really felt the weight of the responsibility.

To everyone's great relief the baby came out crying well— a baby girl. There was blood present within the uterus, indicating a bleed had occurred, and the extra tension this had caused within the uterus could have made it harder to hear the baby's heart beat, although this could also have been due to the baby's position. Sometimes if they lie with their arms and legs in front of their body it shields it, and makes it difficult to hear properly. The heart is just not close enough to where you are trying to listen with the foetal stethoscope through the mother's abdominal wall. Everything ended well in this case, but it wasn't always so.

Apart from me there were just two full time and two part-time staff midwives, and one of the full time ones had started at the same time as me. This was Marion Turnbull. She was older than the rest of us, a grey-haired and nervous looking woman. I never got to find out her background as she was never forthcoming about herself, but no one seemed very sure of her competence. I think they were so short staffed that they couldn't be too selective. Nevertheless she got on well with the routine work and having an extra pair of hands was always useful. There were always at least two midwives on duty, one of which was a sister, so it wasn't really a problem—until one night.

We rotated on to night duty, doing a just a couple of weeks at a time, and of course whenever I was on I always had one of the sisters on with me. The same applied to Marion, until the sister on with her that week went off sick one night at short notice. There was no one else available to work—except me. So Marion and I were to be on together. Although we had both started working there at the same time, she was one of the full-time staff employed by the hospital, not the agency, so she was officially senior to me. However Sister Jarrett wasn't happy. She took me to one side.

'I know Turnbull is officially in charge tonight, but if you are worried about anything do just take over. We will back you up if necessary.'

When we came on duty that evening there was one patient who had just delivered and waiting for a doctor to come to suture her episiotomy. In the other labour room was Judy Payne, in advanced labour with her first baby. There had been some concern about her progress as the baby's head was not down fully within the pelvis, what is known as being 'engaged'. During a first pregnancy the head should move down within the last month. For subsequent pregnancies it should move down as soon as contractions start. Because of this she had been seen by the medical staff, but they thought she should manage to deliver normally, so we should wait and see how she got on in labour.

'You go and keep an eye on the labour ward while I give out the drugs.' Marion told me. 'I'll take over Mrs Payne when I've finished and then you can help the doctor with the suturing.'

This seemed reasonable enough. I went to check on Mrs Payne who was getting really strong contractions. She had had some pethidine earlier but the effect was wearing off, so I started her on gas and air. I palpated her and felt for the position of her baby's head. It was moving down quite well, just about fully engaged. I listened in to the foetal heart and all seemed well. She was beginning to get an urge to push when Marion came to take over, so I left her to it.

Back in the ward I found the doctor had arrived to do the suturing. I went to see that he was all set up, but he wanted to use a different kind of suture to that put out for him, so I had to go back into the other labour room next door to get the kind he wanted. Mrs Payne had just delivered a baby boy, limp and grey and not making any attempt to breathe. Marion was just holding him, cord still attached, not seeming to know what to do.

Thank goodness the doctor was in the next room. I rushed to get him and returned to Marion, who still hadn't done anything. She had to be told three times to cut the cord before I could take the limp and lifeless baby over to the resuscitation equipment. The doctor had a tube down to get oxygen into his lungs in no time. It seemed to take ages, but eventually the baby began to breathe on his own, but still didn't cry and remained limp. We moved him into an incubator to see how he would recover. Mrs Payne was inconsolable. We called her husband who was waiting at home for news, and he came in to try to give her some comfort.

By the morning things still did not look good. Although the baby was breathing he remained limp and unresponsive when handled. He had suffered severe brain damage and a couple of days later he died. However Marion could not really be blamed. Although she hadn't seemed to know what to do, because by chance I had gone in when I did and the doctor was already on the ward, the baby had been resuscitated promptly. But the damage would have already been done. What had happened was that his birth had been too quick. In a baby's skull the bones are not fused together and as the head moves down to become engaged in the pelvis these bones overlap a little, causing some pressure on the brain. Normally this happens slowly giving time to adapt, but in this case the head moved down only shortly before delivery. Then, as the head was delivered, the pressure was suddenly released again and the skull expanded back. This had caused a tear within the brain, which was inevitably fatal. Possibly Marion could have controlled the delivery better, delivering the head more slowly, but the only way this could have been avoided for certain would have been to do a caesarean section, and, as the baby's head had been so slow engaging, perhaps this is what should have happened. But as I have said caesareans were not so readily undertaken then as they are today.

You never know what to expect as a midwife and you have to be prepared for anything. This was the sort of thing we all dreaded—someone unexpectedly losing their precious and longed for baby. Thankfully this was the only such tragedy that occurred during my time working on that unit.

26.

A Staff Midwife

I stayed working through the agency for about six months, gaining both good experience and confidence in myself and my ability as a midwife. But I knew it was time to move on. I couldn't go on working through an agency for ever and would eventually need to find a more permanent job. However I wasn't quite ready to settle down. Two of my friends were taking a break and were off to work their way around the USA. I had managed to save a bit of money, so decided to join them. We had a great time and I stayed there for around five months, the last couple of which were working in a hospital in Tucson, Arizona. I wasn't registered to work as a nurse over there, so was employed as a technician on their Intensive Care Unit responsible for the upkeep of the respirators, although I did help out with much of the nursing as well. But I always knew I would return home to resume work as a midwife.

On return to the UK I began work as a staff midwife at another maternity hospital, a Part 2 midwifery training school that also took student nurses for obstetric experience. After the time away it felt a bit strange suddenly having this responsibility again. I started on the labour ward and, although this was a part 2 training school, they didn't seem to have many pupils and there was no competition for cases. As a result I had plenty of deliveries of my own. When I did have to supervise pupils they were already quite experienced and we always tried to let them do as much as possible on their own initiative in preparation for being on district. However I did not find my work there did much for my confidence. The sister in charge of the labour ward constantly deferred to the medical staff, even to the extent that if a patient needed an internal examination to assess her progress, we should wait for a doctor to come and do it! I was glad when she was off duty and I was on with someone else. I think there must have been some history to this; perhaps something untoward had happened and she had been blamed, but I still felt it went too far, as one instance showed.

Brenda Beasley was admitted from a GP unit because during the birth of her daughter she had suffered a third degree tear. This is serious because, rather than just the skin and muscle of the perineum being damaged, the tear had extended further into the anus (back passage). If it wasn't repaired properly the woman could be left incontinent of faeces. Thankfully a tear as bad as this is rare and I had never come across one before.

The junior houseman on duty was called to admit her. He was still very new to the job and extremely diffident in his work, looking out of his depth much of the time. I wasn't involved as I had been allocated another patient, but I had a competent Part 2 student looking after her, so I didn't have much to do. As I walked down the corridor to go to the office for something I glanced into one of the labour rooms through the small window in the door. I saw one of the student nurses with Mrs Beasley, who had her legs up in stirrups, and the doctor with a suturing trolley at his side as if he was preparing to do the repair himself.

Sister was in her office.

'He's not going to try to do the suturing himself?' I asked.

She just shrugged her shoulders.

'I don't know. It's up to him.'

I couldn't believe it. Surely she wasn't just going to let him. A tear like that needs someone experienced to do the repair to make sure it is successful. Clearly Sister wasn't going to get involved, but I just couldn't leave it at that. So what should I do?

I grabbed a mask and went into the labour room. I said hello to the patient, who hadn't seen me before, then I moved to see what the doctor was doing. I had to be tactful.

'Is it OK if I have a look?' I asked him. 'I haven't seen a third degree tear before.'

So far he had done no more than wash down the area with antiseptic solution and look at the damage.

'What will you do? Will she need a GA for the stitching?' I asked after a brief look.

'I don't know. Are they usually done under GA?'

'Well they were where I did my training, but I don't really know if it's the same here.'

He looked somewhat relieved and moved the trolley away. I left them to go back to my patient.

A few minutes later I passed the office and heard him on the phone to the registrar, who came straight in to see Mrs Beasley, and went on to do the suturing himself with her under a general anaesthetic. She was kept in hospital for the following week and I met her again on the post natal ward. She was still in quite a bit of pain several days later and, although the wound was healing well, it would take a while to settle down completely.

Although most of the time there is a happy outcome to a pregnancy and labour, it is not always so. Because we didn't have the benefit of being able to do scans during pregnancy, if there was anything wrong with the baby it would usually not be apparent until after the baby was born. The first thing a mother asks after being told the sex of her baby is whether it's alright. Sometimes, however, we were forewarned.

When Gail Feltham came to the antenatal clinic pregnant with her first baby, she had already noticed that she was growing larger rather quickly. When examined it was found she had developed hydramnios, which is where a large amount of fluid accumulates in the uterus making it difficult to feel the baby properly on palpation. Although this can occur for no obvious reason, it is often a sign that the baby has something seriously wrong. So she was sent for an X-ray, which revealed the worst. The baby was anencephalic; it had no brain and the top of the skull was missing. A baby with this abnormality cannot live. It would probably be stillborn and even if it did breathe at birth it would not survive for long. She had been given this dreadful news and, after some discussion she decided to come in to have her labour induced. It was preferable to continuing with her pregnancy knowing she was carrying a baby that would not survive, made worse by the extra fluid she was carrying, which was making her quite uncomfortable. Now she would have to go all through labour knowing there would be no baby for her to care for at the end.

I was on duty that day and was assigned to care for her. She had her waters broken and a drip set up with a drug added to stimulate labour. She soon started contracting and I was able to give her extra pain relief to help her. Normally we have to be careful not to give too much of these drugs late in labour because, as well as the mother, they can also make the baby drowsy, which means it can be slow to breathe when it is born. But there were no worries about that in this case. I thought she might not deliver while I was on duty, but by mid afternoon she was fully dilated. It was the first time I had ever delivered such a baby. Sister Jeffs, one of the junior sisters there, came in to help. The baby delivered easily and I handed him to Sister, who took him away to another room. We made no attempt to resuscitate him and I was relieved that he showed no signs of life.

After it was all over Gail was moved to a single room in the post natal ward where she stayed for a couple of nights.

But although she was on her own she would still have been able to hear the other babies, which must have been so hard for her. How soon afterwards should she try to get pregnant again? Was it likely to happen again? These were the questions to which she and her husband wanted answers. We advised her to wait about six months before another pregnancy, but no one could guarantee that the same thing would not happen again.

Anencephaly is clearly incompatible with life, although these babies do very occasionally survive for a short while. Another related defect of the nervous system is when the spinal cord is not enclosed and is only covered with a fluid filled sac. This is known as spina bifida, and I had seen a baby with this once during my training. In this case urgent surgery was needed to protect the spinal cord from damage or infection, although even then there was the possibility of being left with some degree of paralysis. Unfortunately we knew that if a mother gave birth to a baby with either of these conditions, there was an increased chance of her next one having a similar abnormality, so we were not able to reassure Gail that this would not happen again. The cause was a mystery, although there were theories put forward from time to time. It was some years before this mystery was finally solved. It is usually due to a deficiency of a vitamin, folic acid. That is not to say that these women don't always have enough in their diet, but it turns out that some people are unable to absorb it properly. Taking extra doses of the vitamin from very early in pregnancy is usually enough to prevent it happening again.

Strangely enough in the eight months I worked on that unit there were two more anencephalic babies born making a total of three, and I was on duty for them all, delivering another one myself. I suppose it was just coincidental, but I only ever delivered two more over the whole subsequent six years working as a midwife.

On the antenatal ward Angela Louden was another patient I remember well, admitted with raised blood pressure. This settled a bit with bed rest, but was still slightly above normal, so, as she was due in a couple of weeks, it was decided to keep her in hospital until she gave birth. It was her first baby and she was unmarried. All this was nothing out of the ordinary in itself, but what was unusual was that she was a prisoner.

I never found out what she had been convicted of and didn't like to ask her. She was always perfectly polite and obliging with us, although at the same time I felt that she had an underlying anger in her manner. Of course she could not go in with other patients, so she was kept in a side ward where a prison warder stayed with her all the time, day and night. The warders brought in their own sandwich lunches, but we offered them the routine teas and coffees. If they needed a break to go to the toilet, one of us would have to stay in the room with Angela until they returned.

The following week I was back on labour ward, and there was Angela in the first stage of labour. I was allocated to look after her. The warder with her was looking extremely anxious.

'It would happen when I'm on duty,' she said.

She didn't look at all happy about it all, so when Angela was fully dilated and the actual birth imminent, I asked her if she wanted to stay. She shook her head.

'No, I'll wait outside if that's OK.'

I delivered Angela's baby daughter and as soon as it was all done went to tell the warder, who hurried back in to the labour room. I doubt if Angela would have been up to absconding at the time, but you never knew. Eventually she and her baby were transferred together to a prison that had a special unit for mothers and babies.

One of the saddest cases I came across that affected all of us was Tina, a girl with what is now termed 'severe learning difficulties 'and just thirteen years old. No one knew for sure who the father was, and Tina herself didn't seem to understand what was going on or how she became pregnant. She was small, even for her age, and the baby a good size. There was no way she was going to be able to deliver normally, so an elective caesarean section was planned. I was working on the antenatal ward when she was admitted a couple of days before the operation was due, for final assessment and to give her time to get to know some of us. She was such a pretty and affectionate girl, perhaps showing how easily some young man could take advantage of her. Her parents were understandably upset by it all and blamed themselves for not preventing it happening. Perhaps they should have watched her more carefully, but it must have been very difficult to do this continually. Now we all spent as much time as we could with her, explaining what was to happen and telling her there would be a lovely baby at the end, but she just looked at us blankly and we weren't sure how much she understood.

As we got her ready on the morning of her operation we all assured her that she would be alright and we would take very good care of her, but she was clearly terrified and all she could do was to look at us with her large dark eyes and say 'I'm frightened.'

Following her operation, where she was delivered of a baby girl, her recovery was straightforward. She loved her baby daughter, but of course was quite incapable of caring for her in any way. She could never be left alone with her because no one knew what she might do; all she wanted to do was to take her baby from the cot and play with her as if she were a doll. The grandparents were going to bring up the baby as their own and we all felt desperately sorry for them, now with a baby to care for as well as Tina. I hope they were able to get some support for it all.

I remember shortly after this listening to a radio program where they were discussing whether or not a girl similar to Tina with learning difficulties should be allowed to be sterilized when she was incapable of giving her own consent. One of the women speakers argued that the girl should be able to have a child if she wanted to. But, I thought, although she might produce the child, she would never really have it because she would be incapable of giving its care. No one seemed to think about the child. Who was going to have to look after it and raise it? At best its grandmother might take this on, but equally it might have to go into care. It is an extremely difficult dilemma and I wouldn't like to have to make the decision myself, but I thought it was a pity the woman speaker hadn't met Tina, who certainly had not planned to have a baby and was unable to associate the act of sex with the possibility of becoming pregnant anyway.

By now I had worked well over a year as a midwife and felt I had had plenty of good experience, so decided it was time to apply for a sister's post. The extra money would be useful as well! There were no positions available where I was working, so I looked elsewhere, quite glad of a change anyway, and was offered a position as a junior midwifery sister at a small unit near London. That is where I went to work next.

27.

A Midwifery Sister

For the next five years I worked as a hospital midwifery sister. My first post was on a small maternity unit, where we all took turns in our duties in the labour rooms or on the ward, and I enjoyed my time there. Later I worked in a rather larger unit nearer London and I had a good time being able to get into town for shows and exhibitions, but the unit was dreadfully understaffed. I could be alone in the labour ward with as many as three or four women to care for, so I didn't stay long. Finally I moved to a large, modern maternity hospital in Reading, where I remained for over two years.

One big advantage we had in those days was that all hospitals provided accommodation for their staff, which meant that at least you had somewhere to live to start with, and you could take your time looking for somewhere better. I never wanted to live in a nurses' home again. In my previous job I had lived in one for a few weeks. Things were much more flexible than they had been during my training. Anyone could come and go at any time, but I was unfortunate enough to have a room next to a young enrolled nurse, who often came in late and very noisily. Also no rooms had electric sockets—the bedside lamp was wired in directly. This was because the electricity was not considered yours to use. You had heating and lighting, and that was it. But I was determined to use my record player, so bought an adapter for the bulb socket of my lamp and used that. Unfortunately I must have overloaded it because it burnt out and had to be repaired. My record player was carefully stowed in my wardrobe when the electrician came! I was glad when I found a house to share.

Later, when I had a temporary job just before going to Reading, my accommodation was in a house within the hospital grounds, sharing with some half dozen other trained staff. This was January 1974, the time of the three day week, introduced by the Prime Minister Edward Heath to conserve coal supplies, which meant that much of the time there was no electricity supply. But hospitals cannot be without power, so have their own emergency generators. Our house was included in the hospital supply and we were never without heat or light. It seemed very strange when I drove into town and found everything in darkness; no traffic lights and the few shops open were using candle light. Needless to say I remained living there until the strike was over.

To begin with as a junior sister on the small unit most of my work as a midwife continued much as before, just having a bit more responsibility, such as running the unit when on nights. The trend towards hospital births rather than home was continuing with the result that the unit was getting busier. But although by now I felt I was quite experienced, however long you work as a midwife from time to time you will come across something new and unexpected.

One afternoon I was on duty when Trudy Ducker, a large lady, appeared saying she was in labour. She wasn't booked with us and, it turned out, hadn't had any antenatal care.

'I've 'ad four kids already,' she told me. 'Never 'ad no problems with any of them so don't need no doctor.'

She looked as though she was getting strong contractions, so I took her straight to the labour ward. But she was not easy to examine. She weighed at least twenty stone and when I palpated I couldn't feel anything very much at all, although her uterus seemed large. But there was no time to waste. She was already beginning to feel an urge to push and a few minutes later she gave birth to a baby girl. The baby was small, about four and half pounds, so my immediate thought was she must have twins. I cut the cord and handed the baby to Jenny, one of the staff midwives, who had come to help.

In case it was twins I withheld the ergometrine, as this should not be given until the third stage. I felt her uterus, which still seemed large, so I did an internal examination to see if I could feel another baby. To my surprise all I felt was the placenta, already halfway through the cervix, and in a moment it was delivered. I felt her uterus once again. It was still large and didn't feel right. I was about to move away when she looked at me in alarm.

'There's something else coming.'

I looked, only just in time, and a moment later she delivered her second baby girl.

This is not how it is supposed to happen. The placenta of a first twin should not deliver before the second one is born. Identical twins share the same placenta, but if they are non-identical they each have their own, although they are often virtually fused together. This pair was obviously non-identical, so had separate placentae. Even so the first placenta should not separate from the uterus and deliver until after the second baby is born.

Mrs Ducker looked shocked, and none too pleased. With four children at home already, two more was not what she needed. After a couple of days she wanted to go home. The babies were still too small to go so would be with us for a couple of weeks or so longer. But she now had six children, so before she went Sister Hillier, who was the sister in charge of the unit, went to talk to her. Afterwards Sister came out to the office and collapsed in a chair, laughing. Apparently she had discussed the various forms of contraception with Mrs Ducker and given her details of the family planning clinics that she could attend. Then she suggested that in the meantime her husband should use a condom. At that point Mrs Ducker gave a roar of laughter.

'They ain't no use for 'im,' she said. ''He can't get it up can he? Never 'as.'

Her husband had visited her faithfully every day, but who the father (or fathers) of all her children were, goodness knows. She certainly had her hands full so I just hope she did go to one of the clinics for help with contraception.

As nurses we had always been taught to respect a patient's religious beliefs. Of course we didn't have the rich diversity we have today, and the majority of patients were recorded as 'C of E' whether they were regular church goers or not. However I hadn't been in my new post long when a couple wanted to have their baby son circumcised. This operation is not performed routinely under the NHS except for medical reasons, and is normally carried out privately after the mother and baby have gone home, but this couple were keen for it to be done before that as she was staying in for eight days. Sister Hillier arranged for a local Rabbi, who apparently they had used there before, to come in to do the operation. She asked me to go and assist.

'Does it matter that I am not Jewish?' I asked her.

'No, not at all,' she replied. 'You just have to hold the baby and restrain his legs, as he is likely to kick. Afterwards you should take him straight back to his mum and she can give him a feed to settle him down again.'

She assured me that the Rabbi was a good one, as some people who carry out this procedure are not too meticulous when it comes to using sterile procedure. No anaesthetic was to be given, which is quite usual.

The Rabbi arrived, so I collected the baby from his mother and took him into the room we had prepared. I removed his nappy. Although perhaps not as thorough as a trained surgeon, the Rabbi prepared the operation area well, swabbing it down with antiseptic and using a clean towel to cover the baby's body. Then he began, pulling the foreskin forward firmly and swiftly applying a clamp to hold it tight. The baby screamed and I had to restrain his legs. The next moment the Rabbi cut, the baby still screaming. He then drew the remaining skin back and bound it with gauze tape, which he told me should be removed in a couple of days by soaking it off in a bath. It was done.

By now the baby had stopped screaming, but just giving the occasional whimper, his whole body quivering. I put him back in a nappy, wrapped him up and returned with him to his mother.

'He's shaking,' she said, looking shocked as she took him from me and put him to her breast.

'He'll settle down in a minute,' I tried to assure her, although I felt much as she did. I had never felt a baby shake like that before; it must have been so painful. But this is how a circumcision is still very often done and I suppose at least they have no memory of it when they grow up. This was the only time I ever witnessed the procedure.

Another time we had a tragic case where a mother gave birth prematurely to a severely abnormal baby. He was alive at birth, but only just, and there was no hope of him surviving long. The doctor had seen him and confirmed what we already knew; nothing could be done. I had only just come on duty and was still in the office, where Sister Hillier had given the report to hand over to me, when Jenny, the staff midwife who was looking after them, appeared looking anxious.

'She wants him christened,' she said. 'But there's no time to get anyone. He's not going to last.'

I went to the labour ward. She was right, the baby barely breathing, just giving irregular shallow gasps.

'We'll have to do it.' I looked at Jenny. 'Do you want me to?'

She looked relieved and nodded, so I collected the Christening tray, which held a small chalice and water from the office where it was always kept ready.

Anyone can conduct a baptism in an emergency. Ideally it should be someone who has been christened themselves, as I had as a baby, but that isn't essential. So, after a quick word with the mother to confirm it was what she wanted, that is what I did. All you have to do is say the words 'I baptize you in the name of the Father and of the Son and of the Holy Ghost', and at the same time use a drop of water to draw the sign of the cross on the baby's forehead. His mother was calling him John, so I added the name. A few moments later, he died.

June Martin was another woman I remember well. She already had a daughter; a lovely bright child then aged seven. Since giving birth to her daughter she had had two other babies, but both had died suddenly for no apparent reason within the first few of weeks of their lives; cot deaths. Now she was pregnant again and extremely anxious about this new baby.

A decade or so later in cases of cot death suspicion began to be centered more on the mother, largely due to the work of Dr Roy Meadows, now discredited. We rarely had such thoughts then. More recently it has been realized that nursing babies lying on their stomachs increases the incidence of cot death and today all babies should always be laid on their backs. However here, as in all the hospitals I worked, we never laid them on their stomachs, but on their sides, and this is what Mrs Martin had done. Now, because of her history, it was decided that she should stay in hospital for the full ten days following her delivery so that we could keep a careful eye on the baby.

Everything seemed to be going well. The birth of her son was straightforward and normal. In the post-natal ward he soon began to feed well and gained weight. Following the normal practice then all babies stayed in the nursery during the night and staff would feed them as necessary, just taking out those who were being breast fed. In the morning they were wheeled out again to their mothers for their morning feed. One morning when the night nurse went to fetch the baby—he was dead.

Cot deaths are rare, so the chances of three must be extraordinarily low, but the mother couldn't have been involved as she had been nowhere near her son when he died. One possible explanation could be that they all inherited the same rare genetic abnormality making them prone to sudden death. There is much ongoing research into this area but the full causes of cot death are still unclear.

All of this makes it sound as though our work was always depressing and, although times like these were upsetting, most deliveries were normal and the birth of a baby was a welcomed and joyous event. There was Millie Hargreaves, who had twin sons. After they were delivered I went out to the waiting room to her husband, who hadn't wanted to be there at the birth, to give him the good news. I have never seen a husband so delighted. When I took him in to see his wife, all he could say was 'You're a wonderful woman, a wonderful woman.'

Then there was Christmas. We always liked to have a Christmas baby, but it can be quiet then with for some reason a rush coming afterwards for the New Year. This was a pattern we saw repeatedly every year. No routine inductions of labour were done on Christmas day so we would have to wait for someone to arrive in spontaneous labour. One year Lynn Farley came in around mid morning on Christmas day in labour with her second child. She apologized profusely for disturbing us on Christmas morning. However she was in strong labour and delivered within the hour, all normal, no stitches needed, just the ideal birth. She was back in the ward in time for lunch, still apologizing for being a nuisance. We had great difficulty persuading her that we enjoyed having a Christmas baby and her delivery couldn't have been a better one.

28.

Midwifery in the '70s

Moving to the large modern maternity unit was quite a change. Although almost new, it had been built at the end of the sixties when building standards had something to be desired. They had already had to replace the concrete floor in the labour ward when the original began to disintegrate, and some of the windows in the wards let in drafts. Overall, however, it was well designed. The labour ward had ten delivery rooms where women were cared for throughout labour and delivery, and as far as possible every woman in labour had someone with them at all times. Attitudes to husbands had changed and many stayed with their wives, or if they preferred someone else, such as the grandmother or close friend, could be with them instead. Pupil midwives now did a one year course, not split in two parts as when I trained. They conducted most of the deliveries and I soon got used to supervising them. As in my own training, someone had to scrub up with them for their first three cases, and that had to be a sister. There were also a few medical students there for three month stints, but they only needed to do three deliveries each. Their main job on the labour ward was to do any suturing that was needed.

Maternity care was beginning to change. Epidurals and scans were just beginning to be introduced and this hospital had its first CTG machine, the cardiotocograph, which records the foetal heart rate, and with which almost all mothers will be familiar today.

Epidurals were very new and were only available to a few women at first. The aim was that they should be available to every woman who wanted one, but for the time being it depended largely on whether or not a doctor, who had experience of setting them up, was available. I remember one woman who had had a difficult time with the birth of her first child. This time she was admitted in advanced labour, demanding an epidural, which she said she had been promised this time because of her previous experience. But she was already almost fully dilated, so there was just no time to set one up and the baby delivered easily about twenty minutes later. She was still not very pleased with us.

Another woman we had in the antenatal ward was Amy Cartwright. She had been in for couple of weeks with raised blood pressure and had now reached her 37th week. However her latest blood test showed her blood urea had begun to rise. Blood urea is a measure of kidney function and raised levels are a sign of worsening pre-eclampsia. We moved her into a side room near to the labour ward where it was quieter and we could keep a close eye on her. Perhaps, I thought, it would be a good idea to get a recording of the foetal heart, as a continuous recording can give you much more information about the health of the baby than just listening for a minute with a foetal stethoscope.

As we only had one CTG machine it could only be used where it was most needed, so I checked with the labour ward to see if it was available. Needless to say it was in use and I had to wait until later that evening before it was free. After explaining to Mrs Cartwright what I needed to do, I set it up and left it to record for fifteen or so minutes. I hadn't really had any worries about the baby because the heart rate seemed strong and regular whenever I listened. However when I went to look at it I found the recording showed something quite different. A few minutes after the recording started she had had a slight painless contraction. That was nothing unusual as a uterus will undergo occasional, painless, tightening during late pregnancy. However what was alarming was that during the contraction the baby's heart rate dropped from the normal rate of around 140 beats a minute down to below 80 and, what was worse, it didn't rise again to normal for up to a minute afterwards. A few minutes later the same thing happened again, so I left the machine recording while I went to phone the doctor on call.

Although a baby's heart rate may drop a bit during a contraction, it should recover immediately afterward. In this case, as the baby was already being affected, it looked as though it would never cope with the strong contractions of labour. Later that evening they performed a caesarean and her baby daughter, although a bit small, was alive and healthy. I was so thankful it had been possible to do the CTG recording, as without it we might not have realized until too late that the baby was in trouble. She had to spend a while in the special care unit, but was soon well enough to go home with her mother.

We still didn't have an ultrasonic scanner, but they had just acquired one in Oxford, so if anybody really needed one, that was where we sent them. One morning at the last minute I was asked to escort a patient there. It was December and there was already a sprinkling of snow, so I grabbed my cape and set off. Transport was provided by a volunteer driver, a pleasant gentleman, well wrapped up in a sheepskin coat, scarf, hat and gloves. When we got to his car we discovered why. His elderly car had no heating. He had one blanket in the back, but of course I had to give this to the patient. With him driving carefully the journey took over an hour, by which time I was nearly frozen. We were both relieved to get into the warm hospital. The John Radcliffe hospital had only just opened, so was all extremely new. I was amazed to find shopping outlets in the spacious foyer on the way in. It made our hospital seem dated already.

Scans during pregnancy are now routine, but this was the first time I had seen one done and we both found it fascinating. Everything was found to be normal, which was good news for the patient. Then there was the journey back. When the car arrived it turned out there were two more passengers. When it had been booked no one had explained that our patient would have an escort, so now as well as the driver, four of us had to squeeze in. As she was pregnant my patient went in the front with the blanket and I went in the back with the other two. It was cramped, but probably a bit less cold that way. I never had to take a patient again for a scan, but as a result of that anyone going in the future took extra blankets with them. Not long afterwards our hospital acquired its own scanner, making things much easier.

When it came to taking a patient's history you usually only had their own word as to its accuracy. Daisy Bennett was admitted to the antenatal ward with slightly raised blood pressure supposedly at almost thirty six weeks, but when I palpated the baby seemed much larger than expected with the head well down, deeply engaged. Looking at her antenatal record throughout pregnancy she had always been about a month larger than her dated predicted—and there was definitely only one baby there. A couple of days later she went into labour.

'It's too early,' said her anxious husband. 'She still has a whole month to go. Can't you do something to stop it?'

Could she be mistaken with her dates? The baby felt more like full term.

'No, there can't be any mistake. I was away on business for two months, so she can't be due yet.'

We couldn't really say anything to that, so we just tried to reassure him that a baby could survive quite well at thirty six weeks, especially if it was a good size. When her baby son was born he was clearly full term. I don't know if her husband had any suspicions, but nothing more was said.

Another time I was with a pupil looking after a patient in labour with her first baby. She was beginning to get an urge to push, showing that she was nearing the second stage. But when I looked to see if the top of the baby's head was visible yet, I saw that she had a very clear episiotomy scar. She must have had a baby before. I couldn't say anything because her husband was with her, but I pointed it out to my pupil. By now she was fully dilated.

'You had better get scrubbed up ready,' I said told my pupil. 'This one may be quick.'

With a first baby the second stage is usually relatively slow. The tissues take time to stretch up enough to allow the baby's head to pass through and we don't need to scrub up ready until the top of baby's head is well down and clearly visible. But with subsequent labours the second stage is generally very much quicker and we need to get prepared straight away.

I was right. The baby daughter made her appearance, born some ten minutes later. Both parents were delighted and her husband had no idea this was unusually quick for the supposed first baby. I never discovered her true history and no one ever pushed her to try to find out. She may well have had her first child adopted. Whatever had happened she was clearly did not want her husband finding out and we certainly didn't want to jeopardize her marriage in any way, so we all went along with it.

One area where I was lacking in experience was the operating theatre, something I had missed out on during my general nurse training. As a midwife I had often gone into theatre to take the baby during a caesarean section, but that was all. One thing I now had to learn was how to scrub up to assist for the operation. None of the theatre staff covered nights and, when it came to my turn to do night duty, it would be my responsibility. So the next time there was to be an elective caesarean I went in to be shown what to do by Carol, the theatre sister. First she explained how to set everything up and then I had to scrub up to assist with her at my side to tell me what to do. And that was it. The next time I would be on my own. Caesarean sections were still carried out far less frequently than today, but when my turn came for night duty I had to scrub up for several operations. I was never completely sure of myself doing this, made worse because a caesarean at night was usually an emergency, so I had to get everything ready as fast as possible. Often there would only be one auxiliary sent to help and some of them had little experience in theatre, so I would have to explain to them what needed doing as well. Nevertheless I managed without any mishap.

At this time the birth rate was at a record high, a level not seen again until very recently. Here they were running at well over five thousand a year. Virtually all births took place in hospital and there had begun to be a bit of a reaction against this. Some women thought childbirth had become too medicalized and that it should be a natural process. This led to occasional clashes between them and the doctors, with the midwives caught somewhere in between. Of course we all wanted childbirth to be normal, but we had all had experiences where things had gone wrong—and these tend to be the cases that stand out in our memories.

One such patient was Eleanor Grantham, who wanted everything to be as natural as possible. She managed very well during labour, relaxing as much as possible, just using gas and air for pain relief. When it came to the delivery she was determined that she did not want an episiotomy and I went along with this, although she did end up with a small tear. She put her baby son straight to the breast, where he sucked contentedly. Everything seemed fine, but when I went to examine the placenta afterwards my heart sank. A small piece, little more than an inch in diameter, was missing. It isn't always easy to say for certain that a placenta is complete. The membranes that had surrounded the baby before birth can be ragged and the edges of the placenta can be irregularly shaped. The danger is that anything being left within the uterus can cause bleeding later. I informed the doctor on duty who had a look at her, but her uterus was well contracted and her loss normal, so he said to just keep an eye on her for the moment as they were very busy at the time. Everything was fine for about half an hour, by which time she had had her cup of tea and was about to be washed. Then she suddenly started to bleed. It was like turning on a tap; I have never seen anything like it anywhere before or since. She was rushed to theatre where the small piece of placenta was removed manually, during which time she needed eight pints of blood transfused. It was just as well she was in hospital. If she had been at home I don't think even the Flying Squad could have got to her fast enough. But she survived and made a full recovery.

With this being the main maternity unit in the area we were responsible for the Flying Squad. If anyone either on district or in one of the small GP units in the area had any serious difficulty, we would be called out. The calls came through to the labour ward through a dedicated phone line and whoever answered was responsible for contacting the medical staff and calling an ambulance. All the equipment we were likely to need was kept packed and ready for us to take. The most common call was for someone haemorrhaging after a delivery and the only thing we needed to add for this was intravenous fluid and blood for transfusion. One of us would go out with the doctor and I did this a few times. Luckily none of the times I went out were too serious and we were able to deal with them quite easily.

On the post-natal wards most mothers and babies stayed in for just 48 hours, after which they either went home or were transferred to one of the small GP run maternity units nearer to where they lived. Mornings on the ward were taken up with arranging their discharges so as to free up beds for that day's new mothers. Luckily we had excellent ward clerks to assist, otherwise it would have been a nightmare. After that much of our work was helping women with breast feeding. Milk doesn't come in properly until about the third day, and then some women's breasts become uncomfortably engorged for a day or two. I remember one young woman we had who was really in a lot of pain, and it turned out she had breast implants, which seemed to be making things much worse. I don't think any of us had ever come across breast implants before, so it was quite a curiosity, and it would certainly have put me off the idea of having them if I had ever I considered it, which I don't think I ever would have anyway.

With such a fast throughput there was rarely an opportunity to really get to know any of my patients. Only on the antenatal wards did some women have to stay in for any length of time. Here they often needed a good deal of support and encouragement during their stay, especially if they had other children at home from whom they were separated for the first time. But most of the time I was on the labour ward and here there would be new patients every day to care for.

As a result of this after about two and a half years working I felt in need of a fresh challenge. I wasn't sure quite what, but at that time my mother became very ill, dying a short while later. Because of this I had a few weeks break at home with my father, then decided on a real change and obtained a post working on district.

29.

Finally—district again

I was now a district midwife in a cathedral city, working a rota alongside two others, Carol and Wendy. We covered for each other's days off and took turns to be on call in the evenings and at night. Work on the district in the seventies was very different from my time as a pupil midwife some eight years earlier. There were very few home births, but to compensate the local maternity hospital ran what was known as a district bed, a room attached to their labour ward that we could use. We would book women to come in to give birth there with the advantage that we had all the facilities of the hospital available if needed in an emergency. This system meant pupil midwives were able to undertake one or two deliveries during their three months on district, as well as giving us the opportunity to keep our hand in. I always had a pupil allocated to me for their three months district experience, but they never worked alone any more. This meant that, except for on their weekly study day, one of them would be accompanying me in my car. Although only a few were lucky enough to be able to deliver a baby at home, they all seemed to really enjoy their time on district and I enjoyed this teaching aspect of my work.

We had two cars provided to us for our work, so only one of us would have to use our own car on the days when all three of us were on duty. These cars had two way radios linked to the ambulance station, so we could be contacted any time when out on our visits. When any one of us had a patient due to give birth, we always used one of these vehicles. I did enjoy using my own car though, particularly over the long, hot summer of 1976, since it was a convertible.

That car, a Triumph Herald, really came into its own that year!

Most of our work was giving post-natal care at home and we were kept busy with these visits. I loved the work. I was always welcomed into the home and sometimes it felt more like a social visit, especially when I was offered a cup of tea. However sitting and drinking tea with the patient wasn't just wasting time. Often when chatting more casually with the parents they felt able to ask more questions, especially ones they had forgotten or hesitated to ask earlier.

Older brothers and sisters can sometimes feel a bit jealous with all the attention give to the new arrival, so while I was attending to the baby I would always try to involve them in what I was doing if they were around. Only very occasionally were they a bit of a nuisance. A few mothers, when they could see the child was being a nuisance, would just say ineffectively 'you mustn't do that' and the child would just ignore them completely, which could be a bit irritating. However in most cases the children were well behaved and happy to watch, interested to see what was happening to their new baby brother or sister.

The area was relatively well to do, with few of the social problems you can get in large cities, and some of the homes I visited were really beautiful. However there were also a couple of problem areas. One was a council estate built in the early sixties when building standards had much to be desired. Some of the flats were appalling, so cold and damp they even had mould growing on the walls and were impossible to heat properly with no insulation or double glazing. The mothers did their best, but it wasn't ideal for new babies. We also sometimes had to visit travelers, who set up camps near the city. Before they left hospital the staff there always got directions to where they were parked so that we could find them. Their main site was along a wide track quite near the hospital, but the entrance meant wading through thick mud, so I took to keeping a pair of wellington boots in the back of my car for these visits. I would then park the car on the grass verge by the way in and walk the rest of the way, passing small groups of watching children and dogs. They all knew who I had come to see and someone would direct me to where I needed to go. However, although the area looked untidy, with rubbish and other junk lying around, the caravans I visited were always immaculately clean and tidy; I suppose you just have to be organized when living in such a confined space.

All district midwives were attached to different GP practices. I had two practices, but one of them rarely undertook maternity care. With so few home confinements, the GPs felt they didn't get enough experience to keep up to date fully with obstetrics. The doctors in the other practice, however, were keen to continue offering this service. Even so, of the eight pupil midwives I had assigned to me over the course of over two years, only two ever managed to get a home delivery. One of these mothers was Annelies Kellor. She was from Holland where it was still the practice to deliver most babies at home and, as her first baby had been born at home there, she wanted the same for her second. However she lived some twelve miles away from the city and her own GP didn't feel able to undertake her care, so it was arranged for Dr O'Malley, from the practice to which I was attached, to take over.

Over the course of her pregnancy I visited regularly with Ruth, my pupil, to give her antenatal care. When the date she was due approached I made sure I was around on my days off so I wouldn't miss the event. Normally any patient wanting to contact a midwife during evenings and nights would call the ambulance station and they had a list of the midwife on call, but I gave Annelies my home number so she could get me even when I was officially off. She went into labour late one evening and I got her call at about midnight. I phoned Ruth and went to collect her, plus one of the other pupils who was keen to witness a home birth. On arrival at our destination Annelies was progressing well and by 2.30am was nearly six fingers dilated, so I phoned Dr O'Malley, who had said to call him in good time so that he was sure to get there for the birth. By the time he arrived she was almost fully dilated and gave birth to her daughter about half an hour later. Everything had gone beautifully.

I couldn't help but to contrast this with the home deliveries I had conducted as a pupil, not so many years earlier. Then I had generally been entirely on my own. Now there were four of us, me and my pupil who did the delivery, an extra pupil who wanted to see the birth as she was unlikely to get a home delivery herself, and the GP, all present.

Only one other of my pupils ever got to do her own home delivery and I took over one other case, one who had been booked by Wendy but she was away on her days off. I took her pupil with me for the delivery, once again plus another pupil wanting to see a home birth. However there were others who had been booked. One ended up having to be transferred into hospital, although the pupil was able to go with her and she ended up doing the delivery there. The other one was Lily Fine.

Lily was terrified of hospitals and had given birth to all her first three babies at home without any problems. Indeed Wendy knew her well, as she had delivered the last one. Her GP was Dr Phyllis Johns, one of Dr O'Malley's partners, so now, for her fourth pregnancy, she was my patient. Everything seemed normal during her pregnancy and her due date came and passed. When she was a couple of days or so overdue Dr Johns suggested I went to give her an enema, with the hope it would stimulate her labour to begin. However when I went to examine her I found her uterus had become extended with fluid; she had developed hydramnios. Since hydramnios can be a sign that something is wrong with the baby, I called Dr Johns. Lily needed an X-ray—but that entailed a hospital visit. After much persuasion she agreed to come with me if I took her in my car and stayed with her throughout. So that is what we did. Unfortunately our worst fears were confirmed. The baby was anencephalic.

We had to give Lily the news that her baby had no hope of surviving. I took her home and left her with her husband, both distraught at the news. One of their main worries was what they were going to say to their other children, who were expecting a new brother or sister. She had prepared everything so well, the cot with baby clothes all laid out in preparation. But there was still no way she was going to go into hospital for the delivery, so we agreed she could be delivered at home. Since Wendy already knew her, it was decided that we would go together for the birth, rather than take a pupil. The following day we induced her labour by rupturing her membranes. This resulted in a gush of copious liquor and her labour began quickly afterwards. Her baby, when he was born, made no attempt to breathe. Wendy took him from me after I cut the cord. She wrapped him up in a towel to hide his head with just his face was exposed, so that Lily could see him before laying him in the cot. When we eventually finished and Lily was settled we left, taking the baby's body with us to the hospital morgue. We had arranged this beforehand, as we didn't want to have to leave the body behind at home.

There were other mothers who didn't want to give birth in hospital, the ones who wanted to avoid any medical intervention and let childbirth take its natural course – which is what we all liked best, but doesn't always happen.

Indeed I remember one or two mothers who didn't manage a normal delivery becoming really depressed afterwards, thinking themselves failures. Some, however, were really determined to stay at home. Gabrielle Took was one.

Wendy was on duty that evening when she got the call to say a woman was about to give birth at home and didn't have time to get to the hospital. Wendy arrived there very quickly, as it wasn't far from where she lived, but the husband had already delivered the baby girl. Everything was fine, no stitches and the placenta all complete. The ambulance arrived just after Wendy and they were prepared to take mother and baby to the maternity hospital, but Gabrielle had no intention of leaving home, so eventually it was agreed that she could stay. We all rather suspected that she and her husband had deliberately left things too late. She lived very close to the hospital, so could have got there quite quickly if she had really wanted to.

As she was really one of my patients, I did most of her post-natal care. She lived with her husband and other daughter in a rather rundown cottage with only basic facilities. I remember their cat had also recently given birth and six kittens were running about everywhere. They all needed to be found homes and were so pretty that I was very tempted, but had to refuse as I couldn't keep pets in the house I was renting. I made sure Gabriele kept them away from the new baby and used a cat net over the crib, as there is nothing cats like better than a nice warm cot to sleep in.

One evening when I was on I received a call from the hospital to say that a man had just brought in a newborn baby to them. He had arrived with it bundled up in a blanket saying it was his daughter's. What had happened was that his sixteen year old daughter, Clare, had said she was feeling unwell that afternoon and had taken to her room to have a sleep. Later her father had gone up to see how she was. She was still lying down, but there was a whimpering noise coming from beneath the bed, and when he looked he found a small suitcase with a baby boy inside. No one had known she was pregnant and she said afterwards that she hadn't realized either. She had gone through labour and given birth on her own. Not knowing what to do with the baby she had put him, placenta still attached, in the case, too shocked to think any further than that.

Her GP had already been called by her mother and he had been to see her, and now, with the baby being taken care of in hospital, it was decided she should stay at home. Her parents were still in a state of shock when I met them. Clare herself was very quiet. She had a small tear, but her GP didn't want to subject her to having stitches and thought it would heal on its own, which it did subsequently. After that first visit my latest pupil came with me, and she got on very well with Clare, bringing her out of herself a bit, which was good.

It seems amazing that they hadn't suspected anything, but the baby was quite small so it may not have shown too much. Apparently they had thought Clare was putting on a bit of weight, but that was all. Apart from being very cold her baby was none the worse for his experience and, although quite small, continued to do well in the hospital's special care baby unit. However her parents didn't want anyone else to know what had happened, so to account for our daily visits, they told the neighbours that Clare had had a bleed and was very anaemic. This was to be our story if anyone asked about her, although no one ever did.

Then there was what to do with the baby. Their first thoughts were that he should be adopted, but after they all visited him a few times they weren't sure they wanted to be parted from him. Clare was still unable to make any decisions, but wasn't sure how she would manage to cope, not just with caring for him when she was still at school, but with everyone having to know she had had a baby. In the end her elder sister came to the rescue. She lived a few miles away and was married with her own baby. For the time being she would care for Clare's baby as well. That way none of the neighbours would know. How long this arrangement continued I never heard.

Of all the mothers we visited, few had more than two or three children, but Gladys Bamber was expecting her eleventh. She was well known to the other two midwives, as both Carol and Wendy had visited her on many occasions over the years, but now she was my patient. Because of the size of her family she had been allocated two adjacent council houses and my first visit was to chase her up for not attending the hospital's antenatal clinic. I had to pick my way over a broken gate lying on the path to get to her front door, where I was welcomed in. The house was pretty chaotic, but the children all seemed well fed and happy. I completed her antenatal check up. Everything was fine with her pregnancy and I tried to emphasize the importance of attending the clinic. But worse was to come. Shortly after my visit her eldest daughter was murdered. The culprit was a young soldier she had been going out with and he was arrested very quickly, but of course it was all widely publicized in the press. The family was distraught and antenatal clinics were the last thing on Gladys's mind so, together with her GP, we completed her checkups at her home. She eventually delivered another daughter in hospital where she was booked.

The next largest family I visited was quite different. Stephanie Ellin had given birth to number seven when I visited her following her discharge home. She and her husband belonged to a religious sect that didn't believe in contraception of any kind. They lived in a relatively modest three bedroom house and her husband had furnished the children's rooms himself by building bunk beds, using what would otherwise have been the dining room as well as two bedrooms upstairs. They were clearly prepared for more to come. In contrast to Gladys I don't think I ever visited a calmer and more peaceful household. Stephanie seemed completely unflappable. The house was always well ordered without being overly tidy. The other children always appeared happily occupied and welcomed the newest arrival. I often wondered how many more children she would go on to have.

Although there were very few home births we did have the District Room, the next best thing, located in the hospital adjacent to the labour ward, where we could get help if anything untoward occurred during a mother's labour or delivery. It was pleasantly decorated with floral print curtains and counterpane to try to make it look more homely. Lucy Maitland was one of the mothers we booked to give birth there and, together with my pupil midwife, I visited her at home regularly during her pregnancy to give antenatal care. She lived with her husband and Jacob, their three year old son, in a lovely cottage at the edge of the city, old but beautifully modernized. When she was due I told her to contact me as soon as she had any signs of starting labour so as to give us plenty of warning. One morning she called me first thing to say she had had a 'show' and a few niggling contractions. I collected Irene, my pupil then, and we went to visit her at home. We examined her, checked her blood pressure and listened to the baby's heart rate, all normal. She wasn't established in labour, only having contractions every fifteen minutes or so and they were not bothering her at all, so we left her to go and complete our morning visits, saying we would call in again after lunch if we didn't hear from her before then. At midday she called us again to say her contractions were now every four to five minutes and getting stronger. I told her to come into the hospital and Irene and I would meet her there.

Lucy's contractions were getting really strong now, so we started her on gas and air while we examined her. She was six fingers dilated. We sat with her and waited. Her husband had not wanted to be present and he was at home looking after Jacob. Before too long Lucy was ready to push and soon Irene delivered her baby daughter, Emma. I gave Emma to Lucy to hold as Irene delivered the placenta, all complete. Lucy then put her baby to her breast for a few minutes, while I made her a cup of tea.

Next was to weigh Emma, so I brought in the scales so Lucy could watch. Then Irene bathed and dressed the baby ready to go home. Lucy was washed as well and made comfortable. She would be able to go home after six hours had elapsed since giving birth. As Emma had been born at 2.15, they could go at 8.15 that evening, so I arranged for an ambulance to take them then. We had to use an ambulance for anyone going home within less than forty eight hours. In the meantime her husband had come in to stay with her, as her mother was now looking after Jacob.

That evening Irene travelled with them in the ambulance. She would then see that they were all settled at home. I followed in the car a short while later, by which time they were all well settled in, Emma asleep having had another short suck at the breast. Jacob had been introduced to his sister and was looking at her in fascination.

'You know,' said Lucy, 'this time I've felt the baby is really mine.' She explained that she had never been separated from her daughter for a moment, not had her taken away to the nursery to be weighed and bathed. She had been involved the whole way through, just as she would have been if she had given birth at home. We continued to visit every day for the next ten days. Emma fed well from the breast and began to gain weight. When it came to the final visit, I was sorry to say goodbye as we wished her well for the future. But this was what really made our work so fulfilling—not necessarily the more dramatic events that we met on occasions, but when everything is normal and the outcome is a happy, healthy and contented mother and baby.

I loved my work as a district midwife and worked there for over two years, through the long, hot summer of 1976 and the Queen's Silver Jubilee celebrations and street parties in 1977. But could I see myself continuing for many more years to come? I wasn't sure what direction my career should take next. I think I have always been one for new challenges and in the end went for a complete change. I had already been studying with the Open University and now I applied for and was accepted on a full time degree course in biology. It was the start of a new career path for me, to research and to marriage. But however much I enjoyed my later career, I don't think there is ever anything quite the same as the feeling you get when a baby is born; handling a new baby for the first time, seeing the bewildered expression on its face when it has just been thrust from its warm, safe environment of the womb and out into the world. That must be one of the most rewarding parts of being a midwife.

30.

Nursing then and now—some final thoughts

Our training was very different to that of nurses and midwives today, where both are three year degree courses. Then nursing was essentially an apprenticeship, whereby we worked as nurses, learning as we went along through practice and attending lectures. But changes were already in the air. The very first nursing degree courses had just started and there were already plans to make student nurses supernumerary to ward staff so that they could concentrate on learning. Many of us couldn't imagine how it could be done. Where would all the extra trained staff needed to make this possible come from? Where I trained no wards had more than three qualified nurses and some only two, not enough to cover 24 hours a day allowing for days off and holidays. They would also need large numbers of nursing auxiliaries to help with the basic work and at that time we had no more than half a dozen at most, mainly at the annexe.

One of the concerns was that student nurses had too much responsibility, especially when left in charge of wards, and this was stressful for us. I didn't totally go along with this, although of course I couldn't answer for everybody, but everyone I knew seemed to enjoy the responsibility and were proud that we were relied on and trusted so much. Admittedly there were times when I was first left on my own on the wards when I wondered if patients realised that there was just an eighteen year old in charge. But we always knew where to go for help; during the day there would be a trained member of staff alerted on an adjacent ward and at night there were the night sisters. I also felt that if I had only been extra to the ward staff I would have lost much of the what was then known as 'job satisfaction', no longer being an essential part of the workforce.

Then there was the Salmon Report, published shortly after I finished my general nurse training, which led to the abolition of hospital matrons. Matrons had had huge responsibilities including being directly responsible for maintaining nursing and cleaning standards alongside running the hospital. This role had now gone and was replaced by a hierarchy with Chief Nursing Officers at the top, then Principle Nursing Officers, Senior Nursing Officers and Nursing Officers followed by ward sisters and charge nurses. The idea was to create a career structure for nurses in management but, as well as removing many excellent nurses away from the bedside, it in one instant led to the beginning of a mushrooming of paperwork that doesn't seem to have stopped since. This structure has since been modified, and most running of hospitals seems to have been taken over by teams of managers with further reforms currently underway. We didn't have any 'managers' then and at our hospital there was just one Hospital Administrator and a few secretaries. Unfortunately bureaucracy is self-perpetuating.

More recently hospital matrons have been reintroduced in response to public demand. Some people were of the opinion that standards of care had fallen, and this was at least partly attributed to there being no one directly responsible for maintaining nursing standards. In spite of this there are hospitals where standards have still been found to be seriously lacking and no one, not even these 'matrons', seem to be held responsible. Do they do regular ward rounds as they used to? I wasn't aware of ever seeing one during any of my more recent hospital stays, one of three weeks long.

Of course the past can often be viewed through rose tinted spectacles. Our standards were certainly high; both

Matron and the tutors saw to that. Matron or one of her assistants did ward rounds every day, speaking to many of the patients. They missed nothing. Also nurse training schools were attached to hospitals, so the tutors were regular visitors to the wards for practical sessions with students. Then there were clinical instructors, who spent most of their time on wards working with students. They all ensured standards were maintained.

If we ever fell short it was due to pressure of work. There were wards where you seemed to be in a constant rush. Some days I found that for every task I did I was asked to do at least two more. For example if I walked through the ward one patient might ask me for another jug of water and another if I could help them back to bed. As I fetched the water someone else might want something for indigestion and I would notice an IV infusion bag needed changing. As I changed that someone would ask for a bedpan and someone else needed something for pain and another wanted the trolley telephone brought to them. And so it would go on. After I got off duty I would sit down to relax and suddenly remember that I hadn't given the patient what they wanted for indigestion. This would make me feel really guilty and I hoped they had asked someone else when they realised I had forgotten.

In spite of all this most of the older patients especially always seemed so incredibly grateful for anything we did for them. Interestingly it was generally the younger ones who were more demanding. Of course the older generation that we were caring for then were the ones who had lived through two world wars, so they were used to real hardship. Another thing was that the wards were mostly the open Nightingale style, so patients could see us almost all the time—and we could see them, helping us to respond to their needs more promptly. There was always a nurse present in the ward.

That is impossible today where wards consist of small bays of around four beds and this means that as a patient you can go for long periods without seeing a nurse at all, leading some to think they are not doing anything. This is not to say that I think we should go back to the old fashioned open wards.

Today both nurses and midwives in training have to work for a degree. Whereas in the past it was usual for midwives to first train as nurses, midwifery is now usually a separate course, which seems much more sensible, although there are some shorter conversion courses for qualified nurses. Following this change it seems that midwifery has become extremely popular and I gather there can be thirty or more candidates for every place! Seeing there is reported to be a national shortage of midwives there are clearly not enough places.

Given the complexity of modern medicine and the sort of work many nurses go on to do degree courses may well be justified. Nurses have taken over much of the work that used to be the prerogative of junior doctors, allowing medical staff to concentrate on the increasingly complex tests and treatments available today. Some take further training to become Nurse Practitioners in various specialities. They may then run some clinics, such as pre operative assessment that anyone who is scheduled to come in for routine surgery has to attend prior to admission, where they check that you are fit enough to have an anaesthetic. Patient support roles, such as that of the breast cancer care nurses, are areas where nurses have really come into their own, and there are many more examples in different specialities, most of which I am sure I am unaware.

Nursing degree courses have been designed to prepare students for the increasingly technical demands of modern medicine so it's not surprising that these nurses go on to find employment that uses their skills. But not all nursing is highly technical and what it boils down to is that almost all basic nursing is carried out by health care assistants who often have no or very little training, depending on the hospital where they are employed, and no real career structure, although this may be changing soon. In our day we had State Enrolled Nurses (SENs) who helped to fill in the gap, but this training was abolished many years ago in spite of SEN equivalent nurses still being used successfully in many other countries, such as the USA.

I have not worked as a nurse for some thirty years now, but recently have had quite a bit of experience on the receiving end. This has included treatment for cancer and a cerebral aneurysm, and I owe my survival to the excellent treatment and care I received. Whilst in hospital I had plenty of time to observe some of today's nurses; that is in three different hospitals in different towns and cities, and the nurses I came across couldn't have been bettered. But I did witness a couple of incidents involving older patients which I felt could have been better handled, where nurses did not seem to take time to listen and respond to their needs. They seemed to lack the ability to empathize in any way with these patients. The word 'empathy' is one I don't think I ever heard in my training—it was taken for granted. I can remember myself when caring for some of the more seriously ill patients who were completely dependent on us, trying to imagine how it felt for them and thinking one day this could be me. I now know what it is like to feel so completely vulnerable and am just thankful that I have been able to make a full recovery.

However even in my day things were not ideal everywhere and this was highlighted by Barbara Robb in her book 'Sans Everything', (Barbara Robb, *Sans everything: a case to answer*. Nelson, 1967). This report exposed some appalling conditions existing in long term care. It caused quite a scandal at the time, but it seems things are not always so different today. The problems still mostly arise in the care of older patients, an area where there are growing numbers and it is generally hardest to recruit staff.

Some of the incidents reported in the press as having occurred in certain hospitals in recent years are beyond my belief. As always it seems the main problem is too few nurses or midwives, partly due to financial constraints (and too many 'managers'?). Having inadequate numbers of staff leads inevitably to more pressure at work, to such an extent that it can be impossible for them to carry out all their duties properly. They become completely demoralized. Unless this problem is tackled I am afraid there will be yet more problems in the future. Finding a solution is certainly not going to be easy.

Acknowledgements

I would like to thank my husband and friends who have help support me during writing and in proof reading the text of this book. Also my thanks to all the patients I cared for as well as my fellow nurses and midwives without whom I would have nothing to write about.

Printed in Great Britain
by Amazon

27085425R00136